RUNNER'S HIGH

RUNNER'S HIGH

HOW A MOVEMENT OF CANNABIS-FUELED ATHLETES IS CHANGING THE SCIENCE OF SPORTS

JOSIAH HESSE

G. P. PUTNAM'S SONS
NEW YORK

PUTNAM
— EST. 1838 —

G. P. Putnam's Sons
Publishers Since 1838
An imprint of Penguin Random House LLC
penguinrandomhouse.com

Copyright © 2021 by Josiah Hesse

LIBRARY OF CONGRESS CATALOGING-IN-PUBLICATION DATA

Names: Hesse, Josiah, author.
Title: Runner's high : how a movement of cannabis-fueled athletes
   is changing the science of sports / Josiah Hesse.
Description: New York : G. P. Putnam's Sons, 2021. |
   Includes bibliographical references and index.
Identifiers: LCCN 2021023950 (print) | LCCN 2021023951 (ebook) |
   ISBN 9780593191170 (hardcover) | ISBN 9780593191187 (ebook)
Subjects: LCSH: Doping in sports. | Athletes—Drug use. |
   Cannabis. | Sports sciences.
Classification: LCC RC1230.H48 2021 (print) | LCC RC1230 (ebook) |
   DDC 362.29088/796—dc23
LC record available at https://lccn.loc.gov/2021023950
LC ebook record available at https://lccn.loc.gov/2021023951

Printed in the United States of America
1st Printing

Book design by Pauline Neuwirth

To the naked running man, Daniel Landes,
who really should've been in this book.

And to my father, Rick Hesse, who taught
me to question everything.

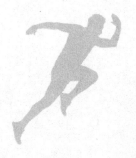

CONTENTS

RUNNER'S
HIGH

A SNOB WAITS IN LINE

Pot is fun.

—Allen Ginsberg

AS THE JOVIAL BRO ANNOUNCES that it's almost time for the race to begin, I can't help but feel a little out of place. Thousands of runners have filled this Denver park on a chilly spring morning in 2015 for the Colfax Marathon, all of us sporting racing bibs, spandex compression tights, and expensively engineered rubber shoes. We're segregated into different groups according to our athletic ability, patiently awaiting our turn like cattle to the slaughter.

We've all paid a decent chunk of money, devoted hundreds of hours in training, and endured near crucifixion-levels of pain (not to mention climbing out of bed at this unholy hour). *And for what?* I ask myself. *Why exactly am I doing this?*

The teenage rebel inside me says that I don't belong here. As a kid, I subscribed to the naive, *Breakfast Club* view of social dynamics, which pegged me as the punk-rock, anti-authority Judd Nelson archetype, or at the very least the squeaky goth girl in heavy eyeliner. Either way, I definitely wasn't Emilio Estevez, the thick-necked jock with daddy issues. I got my ass kicked by people like Emilio in high school, and ever since I've viewed anyone with so much as a gym membership suspiciously.

But all that changed a few years ago. After a decade of hard drinking and smoking, I began running obsessively every day, structuring my entire life around sprinting across mountain trails and through city parks. On this beautiful Denver morning I am in the best shape of my life—a low bar, admittedly—and am about to run a marathon down my favorite street in America while listening to a meticulously curated playlist of my favorite songs.

So what am I so worked up about?

There's a combination of gleeful excitement and stage-fright anxiety surging through all of us as we wait for the air horn to announce the start of the race. The thinnest slice of pink daylight is creeping out of the eastern sky, illuminating the snowcapped Rocky Mountains to the west. A crisp chill in the air is turning our breath to steam as we stock up on as much oxygen as we can before the race begins. Remixes of top 40 radio songs are thudding from nearby speakers the size of my house, punctuated by an announcer—far too chipper for 6:00 a.m.—reading a list of marathon sponsors.

Despite living in Denver for half my life and feeling like I've met nearly all 2.9 million of its population, I don't recognize a single soul here. Everyone I know is still in bed, sleeping off hangovers and ringing ears after a night spent flailing before amplifiers blasting live rock music (its own kind of cardio workout). I accidentally make eye contact with a middle-aged man wearing a Broncos hat and one of those pink shirts proclaiming he's racing for a cure for breast cancer. He gives me a hearty smile and a thumbs-up, and I look away.

I don't want to be rude, but some part of me is just not excited to be here.

Or at least I won't *allow* myself to be excited about being here.

It's a childish, idealistic side of me, to be sure, but it stems from the sincere belief that combining exercise and competition is inherently ridiculous. There are few things in life that bring me as much pleasure as running, but I've resisted the urge to document my running in any numerical way. To me, calculating the data of a run makes as much sense as measuring your heart rate while dancing, or counting your hip thrusts during sex. Running, for me, is about losing myself in the moment; consciousness, time, money, ambition, fear of death—all of it should melt away in the hypnotic rhythm of one step following another.

If you're doing it right.

I've always had a hard time keeping myself in that state whenever numbers enter the picture.* Especially if those numbers are viewed in relation to someone else's, and then suddenly I'm back in high school, unable to jog so much as a lap around the gym as bullies and teachers laugh in disbelief.

Unwarranted defensiveness fuels my criticism of this race and its participants. I'm tired and grumpy, and easily find something to hate about everyone around me. But then I sigh and tell myself to stop being such a snob. These people have just as much right to be here as I do, and who gives a shit if they don't run with the same quasi-spiritual, anti-competition mindset that I do?

And besides, I remind myself, *you have plenty of rebellious heroes who were avid runners. So it's not like there's no cultural precedent for your being here.*

....

* This is somewhat contradicted by the fact that I've meticulously assembled a three-hour playlist for this race, with the BPM of each song curated to match the beat of my footsteps during each phase of the race. If I'm competitive about anything, it's that I have the best playlist of any runner here.

This is true. The sprightly Bob Marley started every morning with a five-mile jog, often followed by hours of soccer games in the afternoon and feverish dancing onstage at night, only to get up and do it again the next morning. (Marley passed this routine on to his son Ziggy, who also doesn't believe in racing or counting miles, once telling *Runner's World* that he didn't even know how long a marathon is.) The Clash frontman Joe Strummer was known to show up, unannounced, to run in various marathons around Europe. The one time he did bother to register, he finished the London Marathon in 3:40, a respectable time considering he hadn't trained and had guzzled a dozen beers the night before. And Alanis Morissette, whose iconic "You Oughta Know" has scored countless runs of mine over the years, regularly competes in trail marathons.

Thinking of Joe Strummer makes me want to tear off this racing bib, throw my Fitbit in the gutter, and just run the whole damn race one block north of the course, as some kind of petulant protest against competition. But for months I've been looking forward to running a whole marathon along Denver's Colfax Avenue, the "wildest, wickedest street in America,"* home to my favorite dive bars, rock clubs, and all-night diners, and nurturing my literary heroes Jack Kerouac and Hunter Thompson (both jocks, I remind myself) during their budding years.

So instead of running away, I saunter to the bathroom.

On the way back to the race, my eye catches a nearby trash can and I notice something peculiar. Mixed in with all the deflated energy gel packets, discarded bottles of Advil, and running salts is a collection of wrappers belonging to a different kind of supplement.

....

* For whatever reason, the city of Denver has proudly adopted this line to describe our most popular street, often ascribing it to *Playboy* despite the magazine never actually saying it. The fact that it would fabricate accusations of debauchery—instead of denying it, the way most cities would—says a lot about why I love Denver.

While the labels of these products advertise flavors like honey and lime, and treats like mints, cookies, and gummies, they also have the acronyms THC and CBD. It's a discreet, seemingly innocuous detail—but it lets consumers know that they're about to ingest a substance that has divided our country for nearly a century.

At the moment, I'm shocked to see these at a marathon.

These products contain the same supplement that got me into running a few years earlier, turning me from a pack-a-day sedentary slug with a drinking problem into an energized antelope who eats 10Ks for breakfast (assuming said breakfast is consumed in the evening, as I, unlike Bob Marley, despise morning runs). And, I will soon learn, my story is not as uncommon as I believe. Not only is this substance consumed by scores of athletes in every field of competition—from the NFL to the NHL, from MMA to the PGA—but it has also fueled my rock running heroes Joe Strummer, Bob (and Ziggy) Marley, and Alanis Morissette.

And, come to think of it, it's the same substance that transformed *The Breakfast Club*'s Emilio Estevez from a bullying, competitive, status-obsessed ball of nerves into a smiling, parkour maniac, screaming with joy as he sprinted and danced around his high school library moments after consuming the plant.

It's cannabis. Pot. Weed. Ganja. And while it's been hailed as a sacred herb, a multifaceted medicine, and a harmless recreant by cultures the world over for thousands of years, it only recently became legal here in Colorado, sparking a multibillion-dollar industry that will soon sweep across the nation, leading to half the US adult population consuming it by the year 2018 (and 68 percent approving of its legalization).

Though right now it's only 2015 and I don't know any of this.

I was planning on discreetly consuming my own cannabis edible once the race began, but I tell myself, *Hey, it's legal now, and apparently you're not the only one with this idea*, and pop a chocolate truffle into my mouth. The wrapper slowly flutters into the trash can, joining its once illicit brethren as I skip back to my place at the starting line.

Back with the other runners, I begin to wonder who else around me is "under the influence." Quite a few, I begin to notice, are sporting the telltale hue of crimson in their eyes—including, to my surprise, the middle-aged man next to me in the Broncos hat. We make eye contact again, and this time I match his bright smile and thumbs-up with my own. At that same moment, a familiar aroma tickles my olfactory nerves. It is the unmistakable musty yet sweet, offensive yet seductive, ancient yet modern smell I'd been noticing on people from all walks of life (from cops and evangelical pastors to hippies and academics) throughout my childhood in Iowa.

Someone in this crowd has recently smoked a joint.

Perhaps I'm not as out of place as I think, I tell myself.

After all, getting high is a pastime that transcends nearly every demographic imaginable. There's no age, race, culture, political or religious affiliation without a strong undercurrent of stoners. (Though it's often only the social dropouts who publicly associate themselves with the plant, leading to wildly inaccurate stereotypes about who uses it and what impact it has on their lives.)

And yet, I'm still surprised it's reached the world of athletics.

In the years ahead, noticing this smell at races (particularly trail races) will be so commonplace for me it'll hardly be noteworthy, but right now, in 2015, I have no idea about the hand-in-glove relationship between pot and sports. I am ignorant to the fact that the natural "runner's high" touted by wellness athletes is actually caused by a type of cannabis that lives within our brains, gifted to us by evolution for the purpose of running down antelopes. I do not yet understand that this internally produced cannabis plays a central role in nearly all our biological functions, and it's being seriously impaired by our modern lifestyle of stress, insomnia, and shitty food—explaining why so many Americans never experience the runner's high and consequently hate exercise.

At the moment, in 2015, I have no idea how wildly popular blending cannabis and exercise is across the world and has been throughout human history, employed not only by athletes looking for a competitive edge or simply to increase the natural pleasure of working out, but also by farmers, fisherman, and workers of all stripes seeking relief from the pain and boredom of physical labor.

Up until this moment, I naively believed that I invented it.

Once my edible kicks in, I feel like Dorothy entering the colorful world of Oz. I abandon all defensive posturing and lean into the camaraderie of the race. Thousands of heads bop in front of and behind me, like one giant sea of rippling waves tumbling down Colfax Avenue. Led Zeppelin's "Immigrant Song" comes on my headphones, and I imagine us as one giant army of Nordic warriors, sprinting toward Valhalla. It's a sensation I experienced often as a boy but lost somewhere along the way. A kind of giddy weightlessness that has nothing to do with health, vanity, or competition, but the simple, mystical joy of *play*.

Euphoric surges of pleasure ripple up my spine.

Gooseflesh spreads across my skin.

Whenever the black hole of exhaustion saps my energy, I make eye contact with whichever runner is closest to me. Seeing that they're in pain too, I suddenly feel a deep sense of companionship with them on this grueling journey toward the finish line. I feel no sense of competition, no need to cross that line an inch before the stranger next to me. *We're all in this together*, I tell myself, and suddenly feel stronger than I did when the race began.

When it's over, I hug every racer who crosses the finish line with me, before popping a CBD edible to aid in the physical recovery that is surely coming (despite the fact that I feel transcendently wonderful right now).

I had initially signed up for the Colfax Marathon as a morbid curiosity. Seeing as I'd been running every day for a few years by then, I'd figured it was time to try a marathon and see what all the fuss was about, certain that I would hate it.

And yet I find myself signing up for my next race that very night.

In the months that follow, I'll discover that a good deal of professional ultramarathon runners—as well as many weekend warriors—are big-time stoners, often carrying vape pens in their pockets as they traverse 50-, 100-, or even 250-mile trail races. When running a Ragnar Relay race, I'll see numerous campsites where bongs, pipes, and joints are passed to teams' runners just before they sprint to the starting line. From recent converts tackling their first 5K to seasoned professionals running the Appalachian Trail, athletes across the globe are seduced by the spiritual, mental, and physical charms of running while stoned.

As a journalist, I find it wildly exciting to discover an avenue of human behavior that is so pervasive yet so underreported. This is basically the coveted recipe of all journalists, and I'm shocked that I am the one to discover it. Why isn't it common knowledge that many of the athletes appearing on TV are, if not stoned in competition (as many are), swapping ice and opioids for edibles and tinctures in their postgame recovery?

Over the next five years, I will obsessively investigate the intersection of cannabis and exercise, tumbling down a rabbit hole of science, history, and athletics—while abandoning my lifelong suspicion toward the wide world of sports.

During this journey, I'll learn that the World Anti-Doping Agency has banned cannabis use by athletes in competition, considering it a "performance-enhancing substance" that "violates the spirit of the sport." This leaves pro athletes risking their sponsorships and careers if they are found with a dirty urinalysis. Many have developed elaborate methods for beating drug tests—or simply stop using a week or two before competition—though hardly a month passes without a story about some promising young athlete losing their career to a marijuana scandal. (Michael Phelps, while harmed by the surfacing of his bong-rip photo, got off easy compared with many others.)

I'll also learn that—despite popular misconceptions—cannabis users are typically more physically fit than their sober counterparts, and exercise more often than those who abstain from the plant.

I will speak with dozens of successful athletes who swear by its power, and scores of previously sick and sedentary people who were able to engage in vigorous exercise for the first time in their lives thanks to cannabis. And yet, at a time when pro athletes are guzzling down opioid painkillers, and 95 percent of Americans can't be bothered to exercise each day, even though it's literally killing them (and killing our nation with health-care costs), cannabis is still considered more dangerous than cocaine by the federal government.

Evolutionary biologists will teach me that cannabis was growing on this planet millions of years before human evolution even began, and once it did, we adapted a complex biological network both to process consumption of the plant and to create some of its properties ourselves. We've been cultivating it since the dawn of civilization (more than ten thousand years ago), and its ability to heal, arouse, inspire, feed, clothe, and balance the human body has been documented throughout history, in nearly every corner of the globe.

From this perspective, the cannabis prohibition of the last century is just a weird flicker in an otherwise uninterrupted romance between man and marijuana. Now that legalization is slowly peeling back the tide of botanical ignorance, humans are being reminded of our storied relationship with cannabis, and its power to not only heal a variety of physical, mental, and spiritual ailments but also to rekindle our natural affection for exercise.

But if cannabis has an energizing effect, where does the lazy-stoner idea come from? Does marijuana cause brain damage, or does it actually *protect* the brain from damage? If we have a natural narcotic dispenser that gets us high when we exercise (i.e., the natural "runner's high"), why do most Americans hate exercising? Is cannabis addictive, or is it a useful aid in addiction recovery? Will pro sports ever drop its ban on cannabis and embrace this lucrative industry the same way they do alcohol (a much more harmful substance), or will cannabis culture just have to create its own sporting events? Does cannabis use by athletes really set a bad example for children? Should athletes even be considered role models in the first place?

Unable to find any comprehensive reporting on the subject, I decided to go ahead and write the book myself.

In *Runner's High*, I detail my efforts to explore this hidden underbelly of athletics, wellness culture, and Western medicine, while meeting some delightful stoner athletes along the way. Like the British man who cycled across three continents and twenty thousand miles while getting stoned every two hours. And the glitter-drenched aerobics instructor puffing on a vape pen while leading the Mary Jane Fonda class. And the diseased and prescription-drug-addicted mother resigned to death before dropping one hundred pounds and climbing out of a wheelchair, thanks to cannabis tinctures. And an Iraq War vet who conquered PTSD and ultramarathons, thanks to his regimen of running stoned alongside a pair of goats.

While I certainly have no qualms discussing my own enchantment with running stoned, and reporting on the scores of others who do the same, I'd like to make it clear that I am not a physician, a fitness expert, or even a cannabis advocate. After spending the first two decades of my life surrounded by televangelists and pyramid-scheme con men in Iowa, I have zero interest in hocking "miracle cure" supplements or self-help programs that promise physical or emotional transformations.

I will provide a chapter with some guidelines for getting high and working out (something I wish I'd had when starting out), but, again, I am not a doctor or a scientist, merely a journalist relaying the experiences of myself and others—along with some data that may explain the chemistry at work behind our experiences.

Ultimately, this is not necessarily a book about weed, or even running. It's about a perspective shift on the whole concept of exercise. It's about engaging our evolutionary reward systems to make exercise as pleasurable as food or sex, and about how cannabis can help jump-start those long-dormant mechanisms.

I encourage anyone with a heart condition and/or who has never exercised to speak with your doctor before attempting anything in this book. This is by no means the definitive, last-word on cannabis athletics. I'm sure in the years ahead, new science and changes in the law and culture will make some aspects of this book appear antiquated, so feel free to be as skeptical and critical of these chapters as you like.

Bottom line: I'm reluctant to claim that running high is 100 percent guaranteed to instantly transform the life of everyone who attempts it.

Though I will proudly admit, it's a lot of fucking fun.

. . . .

BUDTENDER: A dispensary-service employee who guides customers through the cannabis purchasing process, often providing education and recommendations.

CANNABINOID: Compounds within the plant that provide desired effects, like the psychoactive THC and the anti-inflammatory cannabinol (CBD). Humans (and most animals) also produce these internally in the form of endocannabinoids.

DISPENSARY: A store that legally sells cannabis and cannabis products to medical patients and/or recreational customers.

EDIBLES: A food product containing activated cannabis, the potency of which is measured in milligrams of tetrahydrocannabinol (THC).

ENDOCANNABINOID SYSTEM: A biological mechanism that uses endocannabinoids to regulate a vast spectrum of functions—including sleep, mood, body temperature, fertility, appetite, immune system, pain sensation, memory, and many others—with the aim of bringing harmony to the whole body.

FLOWER: Cannabis in its raw (smokable) plant form.

TINCTURE: A liquid form of cannabis, consumed orally.

VAPORIZER: A device that turns raw cannabis (or concentrates) into an inhalable vapor, which is believed to be a healthier alternative to smoking cannabis.

POT MAKES EXERCISE FUN

THE SECRET TREND OF GETTING LIT AND FIT

> Long distance runner, what you standing there for? Get up, get off, get out of the door.
>
> —Grateful Dead, "Fire on the Mountain"

AN OPEN SECRET

It's 2016, six months after the Colfax Marathon, and I think I finally found a sporting event I belong at.

After discovering I perhaps wasn't the only person in the world who enjoyed running high, a quick Google search of the subject revealed there was actually an upcoming gathering of red-eyed athletes in nearby Boulder, Colorado.

Well that was easy, I thought to myself.

Founded by Jim McAlpine—a man who once gobbled a 100-milligram edible before swimming from San Francisco to Alcatraz—the 420 Games seeks to unite all those lonely stoners who thought they were the only ones who liked to blend weed and workout. It's also part of a concerted campaign to rebrand cannabis users as healthy and active, instead of the ubiquitous perception that we're all paralyzed trolls subsisting on 7-Eleven snacks and role-playing video games.* In a few years the 420 Games will blossom into a lucrative corner of the industry, but today, in 2016, it's a simple 4.2-mile "fun run" around the Boulder Reservoir (followed by an avalanche of samples from cannabis companies promoting infused salves, tinctures, and transdermal patches geared toward athletes in need of recovery).

In addition to the 420 Games, the name that keeps popping up in my research is ultramarathon runner Avery Collins.

....

* My apologies to RPG aficionados.

The twenty-five-year-old runner and cannabis enthusiast—known for slaying 100- or even 200-mile footraces across uninhabitable terrain and insane vertical gain—was like catnip to the scores of editors out there looking for clickbait marijuana stories. Ever since Colorado became the first state* to legalize recreational cannabis in 2012, the struggling journalism industry discovered readers were hungry for cannabis stories that went beyond "Just Say No" hysteria. At the same time, few journalists knew anything about the plant, or the culture and science surrounding it, so the reporting often skewed toward novelty over substance.

As the first (nonretired) professional athlete to proudly admit he regularly consumes cannabis—and to be sponsored by newly legal cannabis companies—Avery Collins's phone was blowing up with messages from journalists eager to tell the world about this freak of nature. Nearly every story on him carried the sensationalistic tone of *Can you believe this person exists?!* For most people, Avery's habit of loading up on weed and running up the side of a mountain for thirty-six hours was as inconceivable as an astronaut eating peyote before liftoff.

Admittedly, this is my angle when pitching the story to my editor at *The Guardian*. I'd been reporting on cannabis for years while also pinballing between topics as a freelance journalist (science, arts, politics, crime, economics), but this will be the first time I've come anywhere near a story about sports. I've been an avid runner for three years now, but—even though I had a blast at the Colfax Marathon—I am still very suspicious of the competitive world of pro sports. Part of me is still convinced that the pleasure of running

* While the state of Washington technically legalized recreational cannabis the same night we did in 2012, it took an extra six months to officially launch its recreational market with a handful of poorly supplied dispensaries, by which time Colorado had already become to legal weed what Nevada was to gambling.

conflicts with any documentation of time, distance, or pace—especially when comparing them with other people's numbers. Running is my primal playground, and I have been so protective of this space that I rarely even speak about it to anyone, lest they ruin it with talk of weight-loss goals, Instagram selfies, or, dirtiest of all, *competition*.

My joy in discovering an event full of stoner athletes helps me push through these concerns, and I find myself driving out to Boulder to cover the 420 Games, which featured Avery Collins as its special guest athlete, for *The Guardian*.

Like nearly any other day in Boulder, the sky is clear and sunny, with birds singing and a gentle breeze rustling the prairie grass surrounding the reservoir. While there is no on-site consumption allowed, plumes of smoke escape several of the parked vehicles, and no one is shy about eating edibles or hitting vape pens as they attend a pre-run yoga class.

My editor wants me to frame this as a new fitness trend, and while it's certainly increasing in popularity, I quickly discover the word "trend" isn't appropriate to describe the stoner athletes at the 420 Games. Most of the people I speak with say they've been employing a few bong rips or potent edibles as part of their training regimen for years but had no idea anyone else was doing it. None of them had heard about this on some podcast or blog, unlike barefoot running or parkour, and therefore can't be accused of jumping on a bandwagon.

Though I will eventually learn that, in nearly every sport, cannabis is as commonly consumed as ibuprofen.

I spot Avery Collins at the front of the crowd just before the "fun run" begins, his Nordic blond curls framing a bright, smiling face as he waves to the cheering crowd when his name is announced. Though I lose sight of him once the race begins, and despite being in the front of the pack, I never come close enough to even spot Avery until the run is over. Afterward I try approaching him for an interview, but a thick crowd of fans—many of them young women, likely enthralled by his *Tiger Beat* blue eyes and sharp dimples— have encircled Avery, and I have to wait another two hours for him to meet me at a local brewpub.

Sitting across from him, I quickly realize that Avery is nothing like the thick-necked jocks shouting the word "fag!" while tackling me in the high school locker room so many years ago. With his long, unkempt hair, genuine smile, and snow-bro drawl, he would fit in better at a Burning Man dance party than an ESPN awards show.

Though we share a counterculture connection, it quickly becomes apparent that we're freaked out by each other's lives.

"I rarely leave the mountains, and am almost never in the city," he explains to me, sipping an IPA and watching shoppers pass by on the busy Pearl Street pedestrian mall. "I feel withdrawal if I go more than a few days away from the trails."

Despite being surrounded by the gorgeous Flatiron Mountains, and loaded with trails where some of the best runners in the world train, Boulder, with its 107,000 population is still a little too urban for Avery's taste. Ever since dropping out of college to move to Colorado and become a professional ultrarunner, he and his girlfriend, Sabrina Stanley, an accomplished runner herself, have lived in a trailer home outside the hamlet of Silverton, Colorado, where they maintain a monastic devotion to trail running.

For me, running is the treat I reward myself with at the end of a hard day's work (which mostly involves sitting on my ass and typing). But for Avery, it *is* the work. On an average day he'll spend at least two hours stretching and strength training, followed by another six to eight hours running, most of that on rocky trails and some on an inclined treadmill. Along with the time spent preparing and eating three enormous meals, and another two hours of digitally coaching athletes around the world, followed by ten hours of sleep, there really isn't a minute of Avery's day that isn't devoted to the sport of running—the vast majority of which is done in silent isolation.

Noticing my raised eyebrows, he asks me, "Why, what's your day like?"

While Avery enjoys total isolation for weeks on end, I live in a cooperative house with ten roommates in downtown Denver, and will often have dozens of conversations before I even get to my office, where I edit and manage a small arts and literature magazine. In the afternoon I switch to freelance journalism, where I'll sometimes work until dawn reporting on some political rally or mass shooting, waiting for an editor in London or Australia to give my story a thumbs-up so I can shut down my computer, take an edible, and go for a run.

"Man," he says, staring at me with unblinking eyes, "that stresses me out just hearing about it."

This takes me aback, considering it's coming from a man who regularly, voluntarily, inflicts a transcendent level of physical pain—not to mention psychological torture—on himself, running hundreds of miles with no sleep over the course of days, often powering through injuries, hallucinations, and the paranoia of being lost in the wilderness while surrounded by parasites, predators, and the ominous threat of exposure. And he thinks the life of a writer is stressful?

Avery says he never feels more balance, peace, and safety than during the hours he spends alone scrambling up the side of a mountain. In fact, in the early days of his racing career Avery would push himself to first place not for competitive reasons but merely so he could have the woods all to himself.

"There's no other feeling like it in the world," he tells me, his face lighting up when asked to describe the experience of running in nature. "It's a drug, really. I recently took five months off from running and experienced the darkest depression of my life. Once I started running again, the feeling was *fuuuuuuuucking* unreal. I actually cried, it was so beautiful."

Though this experience does not encapsulate Avery's life as a runner.

Like anyone who decides to turn their passion into a career, Avery found that a whole lot of baggage comes with the privilege. To attract sponsors, Avery (and any professional runner) must maintain vibrant and popular social media accounts. To do that, he must not only be charming, reasonably attractive, and creative in his daily posts but consistently score impressive numbers on multiple races each year. To regularly best the competition, he must be meticulously strategic in his daily training regimens, turning each run into a calculated slog that has the potential to drain every last drop of joy and playfulness out of the experience (thereby eliminating the whole point of turning your passion into a career). Too much of this, and you risk turning ultrarunning into a kind of dystopian, *Hunger Games* torturefest, where you run for days on end just to pay your rent.

"That's where weed comes in," Avery says. "When I'm in training mode, I look at a mountain peak and all I see is numbers: the vertical, the distance, my pace. I don't see anything else, not the trees, the trail, the sky, the animals. But if I take an edible or hit my vape pen, all that glides away, and I'm like, 'Just go fucking run.' Both ends of the spectrum are important, and they need to be balanced."

Avery is quick to point out that his running isn't dependent on weed. He never competes high and often takes extended breaks from it while training (partly due to races increasingly testing runners for cannabis). Though considering he's probably the most famous athlete to actively identify himself with the plant, there's no getting around how large a role it plays in his life as a runner. Also, Avery really, *really* enjoys running high.

"For me, it's like a spiritual experience. Everything is perfect, everything is pure bliss. I'm in the moment, fully tapped into the trail, my body, and am loving every second of it."

This matched what I had heard from others at the 420 Games. Whether they were runners, weightlifters, MMA fighters, or football players, people consistently described the benefits of cannabis when working out. They all expressed an increase in pleasure for the activity, compared with when they'd do it sober. And the more they enjoyed it, the more focused they'd become on it, myopically zeroing in on each curl of the bicep, dribble of the ball, and pronation of the foot as it kisses the dusty ground.

In small doses, cannabis can have an antianxiety effect on an athlete, pushing away the fear of cliff diving, playing a championship game, or continuing to run for another one hundred miles when you don't think you can make it. And then there's the anti-inflammatory properties, allowing athletes to train longer than their sore joints would've previously allowed, and older folks who thought their years of physical activity were behind them to suddenly take up hiking or cycling.

None of them—including myself at this moment—knows why or how cannabis works this way, had ever previously been encouraged to try it, and grew up being told that getting high would turn them into useless couch-monsters.

Outside of myself, whoever was getting high at the Colfax Marathon, and all these weirdos at the 420 Games, I have yet to meet many cannabis athletes. I assume this kind of behavior is limited to the type of people who like to get high during all sorts of activities (movies, conversation, sex) and just happened to realize that it complements exercise as well. So when I ask Avery if he's the only ultrarunner who likes to get high, I'm genuinely shocked when he laughs and says, "Oh, they all do. I'm just the only one who talks about it."

Avery admits he's being hyperbolic when he says *all* trail runners do, but not by much.

"A large number of the elite runners are toking up—I'd say most of them," he says. "It's like if you're about to go to a party, you can be sure there will be alcohol there, right? And if you're going out on a trail with some ultrarunners, there's gonna be some weed smoked. I don't know if that's the case with road running, because that's a different world, and it's still illegal in a lot of places, so people aren't open about it. But I have this experience all the time, and I'm sure you do too, where you know someone for a long time before they admit they're getting high."

I definitely know what he's talking about. Growing up in rural Iowa, I was surrounded by both drugs and religion, and when I eventually abandoned the latter and entered the world of the former as a low-level pot dealer, I was surprised to discover how many evangelical Christians I recognized from church were also hard-core potheads. (The same went for cops, teachers, and politicians as well.)

RUNNING WITH THE DEVIL

My afternoon at the 420 Games and chatting with Avery gives me enough material to stitch together a decent story for *The Guardian*. Though afterward I have a restless sensation in my stomach that I can't seem to shake. Typically when finishing a story, whether it's about wolves being reintroduced to national parks or neural implants that can alter your mood via remote control, I walk away feeling well informed enough to educate an otherwise unfamiliar person on the ins and outs of that particular topic.

When it came to cannabis and fitness, however, I felt lost.

Despite cashing my check for the story and urgently needing to keep that freelance beast fed with new material, I become so endlessly fascinated by the intersection of cannabis and athletics, I find all my work hours being eaten up by the topic (this is the whimsical freedom of freelance life, while the tradeoff is poverty). Over the next four years I assemble a database of hundreds of articles on the science of marijuana and movement, the ever-growing list of athletic stoners getting busted for cannabis (as well as retired athletes confessing their yearslong affair with it), and the explosion of previously sedentary Americans walking into their newly legal dispensary for some edibles, tincture, or vaporizer to consume before hitting the gym.

Arguably, Colorado (and specifically Denver) was central to a lot of the legal and cultural shifts in cannabis happening at the time. Political wizards like Mason Tvert and Brian Vicente, along with many others, helped lead a series of ballot measures to reform cannabis laws—decriminalization, expansion of the medical industry, officially mandating it as the "lowest law-enforcement priority"—before eventually legalizing a recreational industry in 2012.

I must admit, I owe my journalism career to the blind luck of stumbling into cannabis legalization at the perfect time. When I stepped off that Greyhound bus from Iowa to Denver in 2004, I assumed the writing gigs would be eagerly waiting for me. After all, weren't editors on the lookout for high school dropouts with no degree or experience to fill their high-paying jobs in a flourishing industry?

They were not, I soon learned, when they all ignored my pitches.

I had no shortage of passion and could string together a decent sentence, but I was an ignorant farm boy who had never so much as spoken to a real journalist, and was having trouble finding an entry point to the industry. My pitches started landing once I focused on characters like Mason Tvert (who lived and worked down the street from me) and the scrappy campaigns to change pot laws in Colorado. Most legit journalists came from upper-class backgrounds and feared covering the weed beat would harm their reputation. Whereas I was a working-class loner who grew up in the drug culture of an economically impoverished town. I had no reputation to protect.

There were an infinite number of angles to report on cannabis beyond just the changing laws, and I found myself bursting with story ideas and a plethora of editors who were hungry for them. You wanna take edibles with sex-advice columnist Dan Savage and discuss the ethics of bestiality? Sure. You want to attend a Christian stoner Bible study and listen to theories about Jesus using cannabis oil to perform his miracles? Sounds great!

These stories propelled my byline into larger international publications like *Politico*, *Vice*, and *The Guardian* (and gave me a foothold in the industry that allowed me to cover any subject that tickled my itchy curiosity, from science, politics, and crime to religion, art, and sex).

Coping with the stress of freelance life drove me to the classic vices enjoyed by writers throughout history: booze, cigarettes, stimulants (cocaine and Adderall), and shitty food. When I discovered professionally made cannabis edibles (with their measured potency, empowering users for the first time to regulate their dosage and stay in the energizing, euphoric realm of a cannabis high instead of the anxious, lethargic one of large doses), I found that exercise suddenly became a playful, nearly painless activity.

Specifically, it was running (either in the city or on mountain trails) that I fell in love with. It had always been pure misery when forced on me in gym class or fleeing an ass-beating, but somehow running became a profoundly meditative, inspiring, and downright hedonistic activity when seasoned with 10 to 20 milligrams of THC. The experience was so captivating, I gave up all other vices and centered my life on running.

By necessity, I was forced to reevaluate my conception of athletes as homophobic meatheads who threatened my safety.

In time, I found my counterculture heroes in the running world, like hippie dreamboat Steve Prefontaine and Yuki Kawauchi, the performance artist who won big races like the Boston Marathon while dressed in a panda costume or business suit (with dress shoes). Some of my most cherished writers—Malcolm Gladwell, Chuck Klosterman, Haruki Murakami—I discovered, were also runners. As was Stuart Murdoch, the singer of my favorite band, Belle and Sebastian, who wrote poetic odes to the sport like "The Stars of Track and Field" and "The Loneliness of a Middle Distance Runner."

I also learned about Todd Aydelotte, the "Historical Ultrarunner," who organizes 30- to 80-mile races around New York City that follow macabre themes like the Son of Sam murders or the dystopian cult-film *The Warriors*. These runs mostly take place at night, made up of the strange demographic of pop-culture history nerds who also enjoy running an insane number of miles through one of the busiest cities in the world.

All this is what led me to the Colfax Marathon, writing about Avery Collins, and eventually researching the hell out of the intersection of cannabis and exercise. Which, I'm about to discover, is more vast than I ever could've imagined.

IT'S IN THE GAME

"I'd say about eighty-five percent of the NBA [uses cannabis]," former Denver Nuggets power forward Kenyon Martin tells the Bleacher Report.

Martin's interview is part of a 4/20 roundtable discussion about games and ganja, hosted by the sports website. Former tight end for the Dallas Cowboys (and children's book author) Martellus Bennett puts the number around 89 percent for the NFL, and many admit that it enhanced their performance, including fellow Cowboy Sean Smith, who says he smoked "two blunts before every game."

By this point I am aware of the massive spectrum of brain and body functions that cannabis treats, so it's not terribly surprising to me that athletes are using it for a variety of needs. However, I am taken aback that *so many* of them have discovered this trick.

While most football players use cannabis as a pain-management alternative to opioids, such as defensive end Chris Long and wide receiver Calvin Johnson, plenty of athletes are using it during the games, like former Seattle Seahawks wide receiver Percy Harvin, who says he got high before every game to deal with his social anxiety triggered by massive crowds, and former Dallas Cowboys defensive end David Irving, who says, "Every game you saw me in, I was medicated," in an Instagram post where he smokes a blunt before announcing his retirement.

While the wave of pro athletes confessing their love of bud may be inspired by legalization, the intersection of these two activities is far from unprecedented. Throughout the 1970s, NFL star Dave Meggyesy was chairman of the group Jocks for Joynts, which advocated for changes in marijuana policy among sports teams and general awareness of the role cannabis can play in physical activity (the Jocks once challenged an anti-marijuana group to a game of softball, offering to play stoned while they played sober—but the group declined).

Former Philadelphia Flyers enforcer Riley Cote tells me that at least half the players in the National Hockey League (where twenty-eight of the thirty-one teams reside inside in a legalized state or Canadian province) are using cannabis—and if narrowed to only CBD products, that number jumps to around 90 percent. Cote has become an advocate for cannabis use in sports through the organization Athletes for Care. Following pressure from the players' union, Major League Baseball agreed in 2020 to remove cannabis from its list of prohibited substances (while still forbidding its players from being sponsored by a cannabis company or being high in competition).

The Pro Golfers' Association has not been so chill, suspending several players for cannabis use and releasing a statement denouncing CBD after it was reported that at least half the golfers on the PGA senior tour were using the substance.

Over at World Wrestling Entertainment, hard drugs are banned but a "weed tax" of $2,500 is all that's asked of performers caught using cannabis. "That's the thing a lot of people don't know," says WWE wrestler Enzo Amore. "Probably half the locker room smokes pot."

A number of Ultimate Fighting Championship athletes, like Nate Diaz, Elias Theodorou, and Derrick Lewis, proudly confess to getting high. There's even a stoned jiujitsu league, High Rollerz, where fighters share a joint before slamming each other to the mat. "It makes you more in tune with your body," says comedian and MMA commentator Joe Rogan. "You don't get so blitzed that you don't know how to curl your bicep. You get just a *little* high."

Cannabis use has been a staple of the bodybuilding world for decades, as evidenced by Arnold Schwarzenegger smiling as he takes several tokes off a joint in the 1977 documentary *Pumping Iron*.

Ultrarunner (and cannabis enthusiast) Flavie Dokken, who spent years as a bodybuilder before switching to running, explained to me, "It's not uncommon for bodybuilders to push themselves so hard when lifting weights that they puke. Cannabis is excellent for curing nausea and stimulating appetite." Which is important in a sport where you have to eat up to six meals a day, sometimes even waking in the middle of the night to pound some protein.

"I also use it as a replacement for pre-workout or caffeine drinks. A strong sativa will energize me just as well," she adds in her adorable French accent (she grew up in the French Alps before relocating to Colorado). "It helps me to zone in on the workouts."

While she is still relatively new to the sport of ultrarunning, she's already landed a sponsor in Wana Brands, one of the premier cannabis edible companies in Colorado (championed for its fully infused gummies, as opposed to others that merely spray THC on the outside of the candy).

Flavie backs up what Avery Collins says about cannabis in the trail-running community, telling me, "I would say about ninety percent of them are using cannabis, even the athletes who are sponsored, but they have to be hush-hush about it. After races, around the bonfire, everyone passes joints around. It's bigger in trail running than in any other sport. It just goes really well with being in nature, focusing on your surroundings, taking in the scenery."

Like many ultrarunners, Flavie lives and trains in Boulder. While all my punk rock friends in Denver like to make fun of the faux-progressive cartoon world of Boulder's upper-class liberals, we often have great reverence for Boulder's origin story of scrappy hippies attempting to build an artistic utopia.

Like Taos, New Mexico, and Woodstock, New York, Boulder was one of the post–flower power rural enclaves for counterculturists fleeing the idealistic failures of the 1970s, attracting a mix of weirdo writers like Stephen King and Allen Ginsberg alongside the post-California wellness movement of vegans, yogis, organic urban farmers, and psychotropic horticulturalists.

It was a time of hippies looking to "lose the smog" and go "back to the garden," as the Joni Mitchell lyric goes, a time of abandoning the urban life of San Francisco, Los Angeles, and New York and setting up communes in nature, attempting to live as one with the earth—and to enjoy running upon it.

Within this cultural stew came one of the most prominent trail-running communities in the world. After the 1972 Olympic marathon gold medalist Frank Shorter (credited with sparking the running boom of the 1980s) moved to Boulder, a momentum of the very best runners in the world relocating to this once-sleepy Colorado town took hold—and continues to this day. Running for fun was still a weird thing to do in the seventies, so the filthy-looking trail runners, with their tiny shorts, tanned muscles, and dizzy demeanor, fit right in alongside the acid-fried weirdos spinning in circles and reciting lines from *Howl* in the park.

The ideal breeding-ground for cults, Boulder was home to the Divine Madness Running Club, which earned such a pejorative moniker when members began slaying ultramarathons in the 1990s. The team of runners were tackling 130 to 150 miles a week on the mountain trails and scoring big at races like the Leadville Trail 100. Though they certainly lived up to their cultlike reputation. The group's food, money, sleep, workouts, and social and sexual lives were all meticulously mapped out by a man named Yo Tizer—who was later sued by multiple female members of the group for abuse, alongside accusations of sexual assault. In a town of eccentric spiritualists, communes in geodesic domes, and jugglers living in vans down by the river, the Divine Madness Running Club was seen as one of many kooky threads in the Boulder tapestry.

Though surely Boulder's community of counterculture runners was one of those mountain-town eccentricities that didn't exist in the rest of the world, right? All those basic, normal people who engage in moderate exercise for the physical and emotional benefits, naturally they weren't using pot—were they?

SENIORS AND SOCCER MOMS

This was the question on the mind of researcher Angela Bryan, a researcher at the University of Colorado Boulder (CU Boulder) in 2016.

Throughout her career as a health psychologist, Angela had conducted several studies on the potentially negative impacts of cannabis use on children, while simultaneously investigating why Americans weren't exercising and how to change that. Never had she considered the two subjects would overlap until cannabis was legalized in 2012. Angela wondered if an increase in public use could lead to a widespread decrease in exercise and an uptick in obesity (as this was the default assumption many held of the substance at the time). But as she dug into the research, she was surprised to find that cannabis users were less likely to develop type 2 diabetes, and may even be *more* likely to exercise. As legalization transformed Colorado, Angela, her graduate students, and her neuroscientist husband, Kent Hutchison, launched a series of studies looking at the various demographics of people using cannabis and for what purpose.

Despite learning about cannabis use in pro sports, and my own ubiquitous use while running, I was still shocked at the results of her survey on the exercise habits of normal people living in legalized states.

"We found that eighty percent of the six hundred respondents to the survey said they used cannabis before or after working out," Bryan tells me while sitting in her exercise lab at CU Boulder. (A few months from now I'll be getting high and running on a treadmill in this lab for one of her groundbreaking studies.) She also mentions that her research shows that "if you look at data of long-term cannabis users, you see that they have lower body mass index, better waist-to-hip ratio, lower rates of diabetes, and better insulin function."

(Subsequent studies have also revealed that cannabis users are 10 percent less likely to get cancer, and have lower mortality rates when experiencing heart failure, than their sober counterparts.)

All this time I'd assumed that getting high and sprinting through the woods was my own freaky, Gonzo ritual. Learning that ultrarunners and other pro athletes were doing it was surprising but understandable, since these people live in their own bizarre realm of pain and manic determination. But to learn that this tradition was also embraced by the suburban pumpkin-spice crowd? That was a surreal pill to swallow.

Following data showing that seniors were actually the fastest-growing demographic of cannabis users, Angela and Kent began looking at the exercise habits of adults over age sixty and found that those who used cannabis were more healthy and active than those who didn't.

"Older adults staying active into their later years is a great predictor of cognitive function and quality of life," she says. "But the unfortunate reality is, the older we get, the more stuff hurts, making activity difficult. Cannabis can have a role to play in that pain reduction and helping older adults stay active longer. Anecdotally, we've heard of a lot of older adults who've cut the medications they take in half after they begin using cannabis."

A recent study out of the University of California San Diego shows that 15 percent of US seniors are currently using cannabis to treat the symptoms of aging (and it's worth pondering how many were apprehensive to admit such a thing to a pollster and lied).

After returning home from Boulder, I attend a party to celebrate the launch of yet another cannabis magazine in Denver (I think legal weed is almost single-handedly saving the print industry in Colorado) and am introduced to one of these stoner seniors.

Known to the running world as "America's Marathon Man," Jerry Dunn is a seventy-four-year-old ultrarunner and cannabis advocate who is on a mission to change his fellow septuagenarians' views on this sacred plant. Tall, with wispy white hair and a goatee, he looks not unlike present-day Tommy Chong—but with some seriously meaty calves.

"I'm not here to tell anyone to be like me or do what I do," he tells me while sporting a baseball cap that reads JUST SAY YES, his campaign promoting cannabis use for veterans. "I'm just saying to my generation that they should take a look how they're living, how they're thinking, and if they want to change, cannabis has the power to change how you think and live."

While Jerry is proud that he's been using cannabis for the past forty-eight years, it was only recently that he became public about it. Given its illegality and his fame as an accomplished road marathoner (a notably more conservative world than trail running), Jerry kept his cannabis use a secret for most of his adult life. Following legalization, he began broaching the subject with his fellow runners, and he was surprised to find that—just like the Christian stoners sitting in my church, having no idea they weren't the only ones high on Sunday morning—many of his fellow athletes had been getting high during both training and races for years.*

....

* The night before we met, Jerry was having dinner with the director of a very famous trail race, and when Jerry admitted to him that he enjoys cannabis, the race director also

Similar to myself and many stoner athletes I've met, Jerry hated running throughout his teens and twenties—preferring the dizzy mistress of booze and barstools to bongs and bustling. Despite being drafted for the Vietnam War in 1966, Jerry managed to get stationed in Germany instead, where he began his ten-year career as a hardened alcoholic. After serving his time in the military, he drifted down to Florida to manage a restaurant and get as much beach time as possible. With his long legs and slim frame, he was constantly told he looked like a runner and would always reply, "I *hate* running," recalling the drills he was forced to perform in the army.

"So just to get them to shut the fuck up, I ran a half mile with the lifeguards on the beach one day in 1975, and found it was actually a lot of fun."

For the next two years this was the only kind of running Jerry did—for fun, on the beach, with no shoes. Often he'd try it with his eyes closed, early in the morning when the beach was empty, keeping one foot along the shoreline. "Running is inherently a childlike activity," he tells me with a knowing smile. "Kids just go out and run for play, and when I go running, I return to that state of childlike play. A racecourse is really nothing but a big playground."

Jerry had been introduced to cannabis a few years earlier and found that it enhanced that playful mental state when combined with running.

"I didn't get as tired, and the world around me became more vibrant," he says of running high. "I found myself focusing on the natural world around me, rather than thinking about what I've got to do later that day. I'm just out there playing, instead of thinking of it as a training run."

....

confessed to taking an edible before he ran his own courses. Though given his status in the industry and the prohibitions against cannabis use in sport, this person declined to go on the record for this book.

Maintaining a sense of play within training became important for Jerry in the years following, when he began entering races and pushing his body to extremes. Despite being well into his forties, Jerry began running marathons in the 1980s. (He'd given up booze entirely years earlier, as it was getting in the way of his running.) He wasn't interested in serious competition, just in seeing what his body was capable of. When marathons became comfortable enough, he tackled his first 100-mile race in 1989. Two years later, in celebration of the fifteenth anniversary of Habitat for Humanity, he ran and cycled his way from San Francisco to Washington, DC. To celebrate the hundredth anniversary of the Boston Marathon, he ran the entire course every day for twenty-six days leading up to the event. In the year 2000, he attempted to run 200 marathons in a year but only made it to 186.

"I got a lot of attention when I was doing all these crazy things," Jerry tells me the next day, when we go for a run together in Denver's City Park. "But they didn't meet certain standards for the *Guinness Book of World Records*, and then I was like, 'Fuck you—I just wanted to see if I could do this. I'm not doing this for your book.' I never played sports as a kid, and once I got into ultrarunning, all competition went away. I never worried about split times or my pace—never wore one of those smart watches. I just wanted to see how far I could go. I was just running to have a good time."

Like a lot of people, I find Jerry's approach to running inspiring.

He articulates a lot of ideas I've been ruminating on over my (admittedly limited) years as a runner but couldn't quite figure out. I've always assumed sports culture is centered around males ages sixteen to thirty, and exclusively revolves around besting the competition for the entertainment of an audience (most of whom never exercise). But for me and Jerry (and, I will soon learn, scores of others), running is just a weird thing to do in the woods for our own amusement. What any other runner is doing is none of our business.

Both of us were well into our thirties before we ever (voluntarily) exercised and had wildly indulgent, hedonistic lifestyles leading up to that. Neither of us dreamed of winning races or being sponsored when we began running. Not that those things are inherently bad; I just believe they can distract you from the unbridled, in-the-moment playfulness at the core of stoned running.

At the same time, *so many* professional athletes are using cannabis, both in training and competition, and it doesn't seem to be harming their performance by any means (in fact, just the opposite, as we'll get into later). Perhaps it's my own cultural hang-ups about competition—having gone the "turn on, tune in, drop out" route myself years earlier—that clouds my judgment on this topic.

I mean, if I truly believe that pot makes exercise fun, and consider it at odds with competition, then that suggests that competition is incompatible with fun (and therefore incompatible with weed). Is that true? Do I really believe that the nature of competition is inherently toxic and we're all better off ditching our smart watches, deleting our Strava accounts, and just go run (high) alone in the woods?

Or is there something more to competition that I don't currently understand?

Can playfulness and competition coexist inside the same behavior?

Was the trail-running world—with some fiercely competitive events—made up of as many stoners as Avery and Flavie say? And if so, are they having as much fun clashing against one another in the mountains as I have running in Denver parks alone, listening to Black Sabbath and having no idea how far or fast I've gone?

To answer these questions, I'll have to leave the cushy confines of my city-boy life and enter the eternally quiet (yet eerily menacing) world of the Rocky Mountains.

CAN CANNABIS AND COMPETITION COEXIST?

HOW THE CHEERFULLY STONED ARE SMOKING THE TOUGHEST RACES

In long-distance running the only opponent you have to beat is yourself, the way you used to be.

—Haruki Murakami, *What I Talk About When I Talk About Running*

A SPORT OF MISFITS

Following the collapse of the mining industry, Colorado became littered with ghost towns. They'd never known an economy that wasn't centered around hard-drinking laborers, and when the jobs dried up, busy main streets were consumed by nature in a matter of months. Nearly a century later, when the sport of endurance trail running began to take hold in the 1980s, Colorado mountain towns like Leadville, Steamboat Springs, and Silverton—which had barely survived the Great Depression—found a new revenue stream in the form of ultramarathon races.

Much like the lore of miners, it was believed that only the burliest, most determined and desperate souls could traverse these unholy trails for 50, 100, or even 250 miles. This drew some eccentric yet undeniably hardworking athletes to the area. None would be considered "professionals," as there were few sponsorship deals for trail runners at the time. However, these were often highly accomplished individuals with money to spend, and the saloons, brothels, and opium dens that once served miners were now transformed into hot springs, hotels, and microbreweries that gobbled up the expendable income of these travelers. Suddenly a new gold rush was born— one that revolved around medals instead of nuggets.

It's the steep climbs, rocky trails, and insane elevation (around ten thousand feet just at the trailheads) that attract so many ultrarunners to Silverton, Colorado. Even the drive to get there is terrifying. My heart is pounding as I navigate a rented minivan around some of the most treacherous roads I've encountered in my sixteen years as a Coloradan. *The Shining* soundtrack plays on my stereo as I wind around cliffs with no guardrails, knocking a few pieces of gravel over a thousand-foot drop. The engine revs to a piercing screech as I ascend the steep hills, tires squealing as I jerk the wheel around unexpected turns.

For centuries this harsh environment worked to the advantage of the Ute Indians in their fight to keep miners from ravaging their sacred land. One such defeated miner described the area in 1861 as "the highest, roughest, broadest, and most abrupt of all the mountain ranges." (As these stories often go, the natives were eventually crushed by the ruthless march of capitalism.)

Today, Silverton looks nearly the same as it did a century earlier, when it was a gold rush mining town, with its wooden storefronts and unpaved main street. While only 630 people occupy the town, when I visit it's bustling with tourists (mainly from Texas), many of them renting high-powered four-wheelers to go whoop it up on the mountains.

You can imagine how much the trail runners appreciate this.

Many of Silverton's year-round residents belong to the somewhat unflattering moniker of "dirtbag" culture: those whose lives revolve around some combination of running, rock climbing, skiing, snowboarding, hiking, or any of the endless new outdoor recreations invented each year. Many live in domesticated vans half the year, traveling around national and state parks, looking for new ways to explore the fun side of danger. While they're certainly not *all* stoners, cannabis is definitely a central ingredient to the dirtbag world. Which is what brings me to Silverton, home of Avery Collins and his equally accomplished girlfriend, ultrarunner Sabrina Stanley.

Despite living in Denver, I don't get to the mountains all that often.

While most of my friends know me as the farm boy from Iowa, I am very much a city fella. To me, one of the greatest advantages of living in a city is not having to own a car, a privilege I've taken advantage of for the past sixteen years. This makes for a thrifty, low-stress existence, but it also makes it difficult to visit the mountains. Since public transportation from Denver to the mountains was gutted (in favor of highway commerce), I make due with running in the city.

I'm breaking my no-driving streak in part because Silverton is home to the Hardrock 100, an iconic race for any serious ultrarunner, and I'm curious to explore the central nature of dirtbag culture. Throughout the sixties and seventies, when the freaks of Haight-Ashbury and Venice Beach descended on these otherwise conservative mountain towns, the ranchers, cops, and tourism developers often branded them as lazy and useless. And yet they essentially laid the foundation of a fitness movement that became central to the Colorado economy.

Cannabis is now following a similar narrative, going from a source of suspicion and shame to being championed by the mainstream after it proved itself a lucrative commodity. Both cannabis and trail running were once on the fringes of society, and the two go together just as well now as they did then. Though how can that be? How is it that competition and cannabis fit together well enough to create an entire cultural movement that's come to define our state?

After my conversation with Jerry Dunn about the playfully present state of stoned running, I keep thinking about what Avery Collins told me about cannabis allowing him to forget all the numbers of training (calories, elevation, pace) and just run. But he also added that in order to train at an elite level, he'd often take long sabbaticals from cannabis so he could focus on the math.

When he told me about running the Tor des Géants—a 205-mile race with ninety thousand feet of elevation gain through Italy's Aosta Valley—only weeks after being injured in a car accident, resulting in further injuries during the race (two displaced vertebrae, two separated ribs, a few torn tendons in his left foot, and his right ankle popping out of joint—while still finishing in eleventh place), my inevitable question was, *why?*

"If I didn't run that race, I could've lost all my sponsors. And that's the downside of all this. All the time I think how cool it would be to not have sponsors, to just run whenever and wherever I wanted and just be a hippie. But then I'd have to get a job. Whenever I think about that, I tell myself there will eventually be a day when I don't have sponsors."

It's the balance of these two positive and negative currents (playfulness versus ambition) that intrigues me. It's a conundrum I often observed during my years as an arts reporter, seeing creative idealists struggle with the cold realities of building a career and consistently sharpening their skills—when all they wanted to do was get high and follow whatever charmed their heart that particular day.

But is running the same thing as being an artist?

I haven't been in the running world long enough to say (not to mention I don't have many runner friends, and almost exclusively do it alone).

Thankfully, Meghan Hicks, editor of the ultra- and trail-running online magazine *iRunFar*, is also a resident of Silverton. Before meeting up with Avery and Sabrina, I sit down with Meghan in a local park, hoping to learn more about the history and nature of this goofy sport.

As we share a picnic table while drinking cocoa (which she graciously brought from home), Meghan explains that trail running wasn't always such a competitive sport. A century before sponsors, race directors, and feverishly competitive athletes came to define ultramarathons, it used to be just a pleasant weekend stroll through the woods.

"Ultrarunning has its roots in pedestrianism," she explains as I sip her delicious cocoa. "Pedestrianism has been going on here and in Europe for over a hundred years. It was basically a two-day event, where you'd decide how much of those two days you're going to walk or run. And then around forty or fifty years ago, you began seeing true ultraraces pop up with more frequency, like the JFK 50 Mile, and Western States 100-Mile. These were super-small, isolated groups around the country, which grew a little bit each year."

While you can spot casual runners in every corner of the globe today, there were profoundly few of them a half century ago. Just before driving to Silverton, I watch the documentary *Free to Run*, where runners of the 1960s share anecdotes of getting arrested by police, who thought they were running from a crime or were some kind of perverts for running shirtless in little shorts. "There were no more than twelve of us who ran in Central Park at that time, and we all knew each other," says George Hirsch, chairman of the New York Road Runners. "We were considered pretty odd."

A publication like Meghan's would be far from necessary back then, since there were so few races and any runner curious about another's time could simply call them up for a chat. Today, there are dozens of magazines devoted to both road and trail running, though many of them exist only to churn out native advertising for shoe companies and expensive races. I was drawn to *iRunFar* for its journalistic grit, operating as a medium for hard-core fans and not as a moneymaking operation for sponsors and race directors—which has come to infect and mutate the sport of ultrarunning.

"Today we have a lot of young professional athletes who are getting paid just to run, and that wasn't the case ten or fifteen years ago," she says. "A lot of that began to change when *Born to Run* became a bestseller in 2009, and we all got barefoot running shoes and started chatting with other runners on the Internet."

Following the explosion of *Born to Run*,* Christopher McDougall's book about the mysterious, cave-dwelling Tarahumara runners of Mexico, who slaughtered 200-mile races while wearing very basic sandals, bigger and more expensive races began popping up around the nation, and along with them an industry of specialized gear, coaches, supplements, training apps, and an endless stream of books about diet, strength training, and mental fitness for runners. An unintended consequence of all this capitalism is both road and trail running becoming a recreation of the white middle- and upper-class (a similar fate has befallen the legal cannabis industry), despite its egalitarian origins and simplistic nature.

This is more the case with road running than with trail running, which may be due to the fact that road running is older and more popular and can be done nearly anywhere. While trail running has exploded in the last decade, big road marathons like those in Boston and New York offer more money, fame, and career stability to the winners than ultras or trail races. Which makes for a more intensely myopic kind of competition, and a lot less room for playfulness (in my opinion).

Though Meghan tells me that the spirit of introspective running is still alive today.

"I'd say maybe half of all trail runners don't give two shits what any other runner is doing," she tells me. "They care about improving themselves, doing the run they want to do. Of course you want your best to be better than others', but it's not cutthroat like other sports.

....

* Multiple runners from *Born to Run* have since come out of the cannabis closet, and predictably there's now a CBD drink for athletes that bears the moniker.

In trail running you're competing *with* others, like, let's work really hard *together* and see who has a little more at the end. You want to bring out the best in everyone, not destroy them."

This makes me think of something Barkley Marathons founder Gary Cantrell says in a documentary about his race: "There's a camaraderie to competition. There's a closeness between people you compete with." (Though I'm still quite dubious about the virtues of competition.)

Meghan is quick to add that there are plenty of carefree road runners who do it for their own personal fun, and plenty of anal, regimented trail runners who stick to an intense schedule and show up to win on race day. There's no single trail-running archetype, she says.

At the same time, Meghan adds that "trail running is a sport that attracts a lot of misfits and has a strong countercultural thread." And not a few of them enjoy their cannabis—a substance not known to inspire the mindset of a dominating jock. "When I first got into the sport, it was assumed a lot of people were using it, but nobody talked about it. That's slowly changing, but a lot of the elite runners are quiet about it—except for Avery. It's a tool in your toolbox that can help you perform, and it's a very popular tool. Just earlier today I found a pen vaporizer lying beside the trail during my morning run."

Despite cannabis's ban in competition for being a performance-enhancing substance (more on this later), and a significant amount of pushback from conservative runners still living in Ronald Reagan's America, the sport of ultraracing has developed a global reputation as a pastime of stoners, which many see as conflicting with the nature of competitive sports.

"There's definitely a stereotype in Europe that American trail- and ultrarunners are just a bunch of hippies who are all smoking dope before races," Meghan says. "But there are plenty of European runners who are also getting high. It's just not as acceptable to admit it over there as it is here, because here it's legal."

ALL AROUND THE WORLD

While ultrarunning may have started in the United States, Europeans quickly adopted the sport as their own and built an industry that eclipses ours. Most of this boils down to them having more fans than we do. While a decent number of Americans will participate in a marathon, there aren't a lot of marathon spectators relative to other sports (I know a lot of people come out for the Boston Marathon, but it's nothing compared with how many Americans watch the Super Bowl). Whereas across the pond, fans of all ages and backgrounds attend cycling and footraces with as much sports-fan intensity as college football fans over here. When Avery Collins first visited Europe for Tor des Géants, he was surprised to find himself signing autographs for star-struck kids who'd waited in the rain to see him race.

The "pedestrianism" sport that Meghan referred to really began— and continues—in Europe, where hiking mountains or simply walking through town is a centuries-old pastime. In the UK, pedestrians have the legal right to walk through just about anywhere, even through a great deal of private land. This couldn't be more different from the United States, where most cities don't allow foot traffic for more than a couple of miles in any direction before you encounter a busy highway. Many Americans I know will go weeks without walking more than a few hundred steps in a day.

The European pedestrian tradition of walking long distances, often through a natural setting, is the perfect breeding ground for a subculture of stoned athletics.

Just before coming to Silverton, I came across the *Healthy Stoner* blog, which was created by the British cyclist Roger Boyd, primarily to document his two-year adventure bicycling over 19,000 miles across Europe, India, Australia, Nepal, and New Zealand—all while getting stoned every few hours.

"This is my lifestyle—and a lot of other people's in Europe—and I wanted to show the world that," Roger tells me over Skype as I sit in a Silverton coffee shop after finishing my interview with Meghan. "The UK media definitely demonizes cannabis and the people who use it. So I wanted to show them there are a lot of people who use cannabis and are active."

Like Angela Bryan at CU Boulder, researchers in Europe are beginning to pick up on the fact that cannabis is becoming a cultural staple of sports. A 2005 study out of the University of the Mediterranean showed that 20 percent of French student athletes were using cannabis in their training to increase performance, and of all the positive drug tests for pro athletes, 25 percent of them were for cannabis. This was Roger Boyd's experience during his ride across France. "I met loads of stoner skiers in France," he tells me. "You know speed riding—where you ski off the side of a mountain with a parachute, then glide back down, hit the ground, and ski some more. Those guys love their weed."

As his travels continued though, Roger realized the trend wasn't just relegated to adrenaline junkies.

"Pretty much everyone I met had some story about how they like to run high or go hiking stoned—that's a big thing people like to do," he says. "When I created *Healthy Stoner*, the name wasn't in reference to just me but all the people who like to get high and be active."

Growing up in Hampshire, Roger had always enjoyed cycling, and even competed a bit representing Basingstoke and Mid Hants Athletic Club. But it wasn't until he discovered cannabis that cycling transformed into an idyllic solo adventure (absent any competitor), riding his bike around the English countryside, listening to nineties grunge on his headphones. "It elevated me above the discomfort of cycling, and I found I could go much farther. The euphoric effects of both the weed and the exercise came together, and I didn't want to stop. Felt like I could carry on forever. That was when I realized I wanted to cycle around the world."

It's noteworthy to me that Roger never considered monetizing his newfound passion by seeking out sponsors and entering big cycling races. He just wanted to ride his bike around the world—or to see if he could—which speaks to the whimsical influence of cannabis on an athlete's mindset.

Unlike Forrest Gump, Roger wasn't able to sprint out his front door and travel the world. It took a couple of years of saving, and a lot of logistical planning, but in 2015 he headed out with a backpack, a vaporizer (he never smokes), and a bicycle. It would be two years before he saw home again. Biking around six to eight hours a day, Roger was able to tackle an average of around seventy miles before collapsing in his tent or at the home of some gracious stranger. Many of the roads held treacherous terrain, wild animals, and chaotic traffic, but Roger Boyd just smiled and rolled with it, living the adventure he'd dreamed about for years.

Knowing how difficult it can be to find weed in a foreign land with no dispensaries, I was surprised to hear that Roger had little trouble scoring everywhere he went. "It's everywhere, isn't it?" he said. "It's certainly in every European country. India has a big weed culture—you can see people smoking chillums next to the road. I didn't go to the Middle East though. There's definitely weed there, but it's not for tourists, and you can get in big trouble if you get caught."

There were occasional dry spells, mostly due to the fact that Roger would dump his stash and clean his vaporizer before crossing each border, then would have to try to score again on the other side. "You just gotta find people who look cool, ask them, and they'll point you in the right direction," he said. "Some Moroccan guy sold me some hash he'd smuggled up his bum. It really smelled like shit, but after a good wash, the hash was terrific."

Currently Roger is dreaming up a cycle trip across North America so that he can visit the numerous dispensaries across Canada and several US states—where you not only don't have to wash feces off your products, but you can also be (relatively) sure they weren't grown with harmful pesticides; never bricked and molded in transport; and have no association with guns, other drugs, or any kind of criminal activity.

After my interview with Roger, I visit one of Silverton's three dispensaries, buying an edible and some flower I'll consume in the van later that night (don't tell the rental agency!). The whole transaction takes only a few minutes, and as I'm handing over my debit card, I think of Roger Boyd and his shit-stained hash. People all around the world go to such great efforts, and at such risk, to acquire something we can purchase for a few bucks around the corner. Or in Meghan Hicks's experience, find littered on a mountain trail.

I also think about the UK media pegging all stoners as lazy idiots, and the European race directors who think it's only American runners who get high. In more enlightened corners of the United States, we left those stereotypes behind years ago, because—similar to abandoning gay stereotypes after we legalized same-sex marriage and learned that queer people exist in every culture—once it became acceptable to admit you liked to get high, people from all different walks of life began admitting they'd been doing it for years.

Though the fact that the premise of this book still seems ridiculous to a lot of Americans, typically those in states without legalization (several New York publishers scoffed or were even angered when reading the proposal), illustrates that we still have a long way to go in understanding who consumes cannabis and for what purpose. As long as it remains an underground activity, anyone aboveground will have no idea how many active, healthy, ambitious people are regularly using cannabis.

If more elite athletes were, like Avery Collins, honest about their cannabis use, that would likely change. Though, as I was about to find out, Avery's openness about his herbal habits comes at a great price to his reputation and opportunities.

PLAY TO WIN

I feel like I'm inside an Irish Spring commercial.

I ate a 10-milligram gummy just before Avery Collins and Sabrina Stanley knocked on my window this morning (in true dirtbag fashion, I camped inside my van at the trailhead), and it's kicking in now as we hike up a trail outside Silverton. The sky is overcast, with a light drizzle of rain misting down on us, keeping our aerobic bodies cool. Wispy plumes of clouds surround each mountain peak like erupting volcanoes, then lazily drift across our trail, engulfing us in a heavy mist.

The air in Denver is some of the most polluted in the world (primarily due to a population explosion and gridlocked traffic, caused, in part, by cannabis legalization). The air here in Silverton is so clean, so humidly fresh and cool, that I find myself pulling long, satisfying gusts into my thirsty lungs.

It's been raining for weeks in Silverton, and wildflowers are in bloom all around us. We drink from waterfalls and creeks, sharing the icy-cold water with a pair of coyotes lapping up their own hydration downstream. I am pleasantly stoned and would love to silently trot along this trail, letting my eyes and ears soak up all the idyllic beauty around me. But the resemblance of this to the English countryside is making me think of Roger Boyd and his discovery of the simple pleasure of riding a bike while stoned.

What role did competition play in his 19,000-mile bike ride?

I never asked him about this, but I can't imagine how it would ever be a factor. He didn't seem to be doing it to prove anything to anyone or to beat any records. Jerry Dunn had described abandoning competition, smart watches, and getting his name in *Guinness Book of World Records* as an abandoning of the ego. This implies that competition is all about elevating yourself above others for some narcissistic glorification. And the whole idea behind adding cannabis to exercise—at least for me—is abandoning all that shit and staying in the present moment, in your own body and not concerned with anyone else's.

"They tell you pot-smoking makes you unmotivated, which is a lie," stand-up comic Bill Hicks once said. "When you're high, you can do everything you normally do just as well—you just realize that it's not worth the fucking effort. There is a difference."

Cannabis helped me view exercise as something beyond—or even completely unrelated to—competition. I wanted to run all the time but, as Meghan Hicks said about many trail runners, I couldn't give a shit what any other runner was doing.

I think this is what a lot of my punk rock friends have never understood about my running, and is the same thing keeping a lot of people from ever entering a gym: fitness can be a beautiful, euphoric form of communing with one's own body if you can just stop comparing your own pace, reps, and waistline to everyone else's and move your consciousness inward for a bit. Which is exactly what cannabis is best at (as long as you don't take too much).

At the same time, I'm certainly guilty of comparing myself with Sabrina and Avery.

With their identical Scandinavian cuteness, they look like they could be brother and sister instead of boyfriend and girlfriend. As we hike through all these wildflowers and this bright-green prairie grass, to my stoned mind they look like an adorable von Trapp couple who belong on some Swiss Miss cocoa marketing, selling the image of youth, beauty, and energy. (This hallucination is brought to you by Wana gummies.)

Not only are they both as young, muscled, and sprightly as you can imagine, but they're also two of the fiercest ultrarunners in the sport. In 2017 Sabrina Stanley—with her long, flowing blond hair, sparkly blue eyes, and bright smile—took third place at the Western States 100 (basically the Super Bowl of US ultrarunning), and a few weeks after our hike she'll set the record for the Nolan's 14, a 100-mile run traversing fourteen different 14,000-foot mountain peaks.

"Sabrina has a determination unlike anything I've ever seen," Avery told me during an earlier conversation. "Whenever we do heat training in the sauna, she can stay in there so much longer than I can. Not because she feels less pain—she just refuses to quit."

Growing up in a Catholic family in rural Washington with four older brothers, Sabrina was immersed in competition. "My parents were supercompetitive," she says. "All my dad ever cared about was sports. We played every sport imaginable and were always trying to see who could do something the fastest, the best. It was drilled into us that we had to be the best at whatever we did."

That fierce competitive streak still burns within her, which at times is unsettling to other trail runners who don't expect such energy from a woman. "I was doing an interview after Western States and said, 'My strategy was just to hunt down the next headlamp,' and afterward I got a lot of comments, saying they've never heard a female ultrarunner talk like that. It's supposed to be all kumbaya, everyone's best friends—especially women. I feel like men can get away with that language more than women. I hear Avery say things that if I said, I'd be called a 'bitch.' . . . But if I'm in a race, I'm there to win. After all, this is my income, my career. If I want to have fun, I'd just go run by myself."

Despite my misgivings about competition, it seems unfair that Sabrina shouldn't be allowed to exert the same dominating energy as men. When she says she doesn't follow other runners on social media, doesn't cheer them on or want to be their friend—because "I don't want to be friends with the competition"—I'm a little taken aback. But then she adds, "I don't want to see someone else's work-out, someone else's accomplishment, and start comparing it to my own," and I realize she's not a sociopath, just someone who knows her own mind and is taking proactive steps to stay in a good head-space.

Besides, I've only just met Sabrina, and from what I can tell, she's a very nice person (so long as you're not racing against her), and I don't feel right labeling her as a competition-obsessed psycho just because we have a different approach to running. Also, as we hike, she's cracking jokes, skipping over creeks, and playing with her black Lab, Sable, so it's not like she's without a frisky spirit.

Meanwhile, we've only gone a couple of miles up the trail, and I'm seriously dying.

The path we're traversing is a section of the Hardrock 100, one of the most technically challenging ultraraces in America. We've hardly run at all because the incline is so steep, it makes more sense to walk (though I get the feeling that Avery and Sabrina could easily gazelle their way to the peak without breaking a sweat). I look down at my watch and see my heart rate is maxed out at 175 bpm.

Out of curiosity I ask Avery where his heart rate is at.

"You've gotta be fucking kidding me!" I say when he tells me he's at 80 bpm. "How is that even possible? That's my rate when I shuffle to the bathroom at night."

"Well, for one, we live at elevation," he explains to me, "which increases your red blood cell count, bringing more oxygen to your muscles. You can get the same benefit in Denver with saunas or any kind of high-heat therapy."

I understand there's a hell of a lot more than just our different addresses creating this disparity of heart rate (most notably that these two run up mountains every day while I sit at a desk typing sassy essays), but this little nugget of info tickles my curiosity. Avery, Sabrina, and I spend the next hour chatting about heart-rate training, nose breathing, high-fat versus high-carb diets, sprints versus slow runs, proper gait, pronation, and the galaxy of different running shoes for different occasions.

For years I've actively avoided any kind of left-brain strategizing in my running, preferring to keep it a casual, impulsive activity, never measuring my distance or setting any kind of goals for fear of draining all the fun out of it.

All this talk of strength training and establishing a cardio base never stresses me out or makes me feel pressured though, in part because I am very high and am in a state of pleasant curiosity, but also because, unlike these two, running is not my job. I have the luxury of not feeling competitive about running because my paycheck isn't determined by my being faster than the next guy.

At the same time, I find myself wanting an 80 bpm heart rate while scaling up a mountain. I want to look back at the end of a 50- or 100-mile course and know that my legs just *owned* that trail (or at least survived it). I want the rippled abs and swollen calves of Avery and Sabrina, not to wow my Instagram followers but to be able to whimsically tackle an eight-hour run through the city. I want a more powerful body to play in, but I am beginning to understand that it's going to take a lot more than playfulness to get there.

I'm not sure if any of this qualifies as competition.

I have no interest in besting Avery or Sabrina; I just want what they have.

Then again, would they have what they have without that fierce competitive spirit? I suddenly realize how naive I've been on this issue. I've held on to the erroneous idea that artists are somehow superior to athletes because they're free of competition, but there's plenty of competition in the arts. You could even argue that artists are just as dependent on competition as athletes.

Even the most casual glance at the musical renaissance of the 1960s reveals an intense level of competition between songwriters. Brian Wilson happily admits that the driving force behind the Beach Boys' *Pet Sounds* album was creating something superior to the Beatles' *Rubber Soul*, and in turn Paul McCartney has said the same about trying to best *Pet Sounds* with *Sgt. Pepper* the following year.

And both were playfully stoned the entire time.

It wasn't a coincidence that the greatest songwriters in modern history were all part of the same 1960s generation. They were great because they challenged one another to be great. This reminds me of what Nike cofounder and running coach Bill Bowerman told his team at the 1972 Munich Olympics (or at least Donald Sutherland does while playing him in *Without Limits*): "*Citius. Altius. Fortius.* It means 'Faster. Higher. Stronger.' It's been the motto for the Olympics for the last 2,500 years. But it doesn't mean faster, higher, and stronger than who you are competing against. Just Faster. Higher. Stronger."

Still, I believe a sense of play is integral to achieving this greatness.

And that the insecurity and fear driving a lot of competitive athletes (or just any competitive person in general) is the greatest threat to entering that state of playful flow. Though without the yang of ambition to the yin of play, there is no greatness achieved—and often it takes the challenge of a hungry competitor to bring that greatness out of you. (In a few months, I will be taught this lesson when racing a pair of twin goats up a mountain.)

Like Avery said, it's always about balance. That's one of the reasons he takes a break from the dreamy (stoned) type of running while training for a big race—and never consumes pot during competition.

"To race high would take the edge off, I'd think," Sabrina says, adding that you often need that edge to navigate what is a very complex and demanding task. "To do a hundred-mile race, you need to be very focused. You need to know where the other runners are. You can't be in la-la land. At the beginning of the race, you have to go crazy slow and conserve your energy, even if your body can go faster. When you're running high and in that flow, you may not hold the reins back. And at every aid station you have a huge agenda—tend to your blisters, take salt tabs, fill up your water, eat an energy gel—and if you forget anything, it's another five hours to the next aid station, and you're gonna bonk hard."

While I'm defensive at the suggestion that high runners can't focus, I can relate to this. Shortly after I discovered running high, someone invited me to join their soccer game, and despite having never played, I thought it would be sensible to get high beforehand. Big mistake. These were serious soccer players, and they were profoundly annoyed when I kicked the ball in the wrong direction, forgot what team I was on, or stared blankly when esoteric phrases like "Track back!" or "Narrow the angles!" were shouted at me.

The lesson: don't try new things stoned.

Though just as too much play can make you sloppy, too much neurotic focus can be just as detrimental. Something I've consistently heard from all the runners I've spoken with is that ultramarathon running is much more of a mental game than a physical one (Avery goes so far as to say it's 90 percent mental). Look at any ultraracing documentary and you'll see the runners' aid station crew spending more time on nursing runners' psychological wounds than physical ones, acting more like therapists than physicians.

"When you haven't slept in a few days, and you still have twenty or thirty miles to go, you can really lose it," Avery says. After a certain point, the battle moves from your legs to your head, and you have to do all sorts of psychological maneuvering to get it back on track.

For some people, this looks like a job for weed.

"It's an open secret that all the biggest names in the sport are carrying vape pens during races and getting high, which I don't condone," Sabrina says, adding that she doesn't use cannabis herself.

It does make sense that a little puff off a vape pen (which generally produces a much milder intoxication than smoke or an edible) would help return a mind to a state of playful joy when you're thirty-six hours into a grueling mountain race and aren't sure you can handle another peak. Losing your confidence when facing a challenge can annihilate a runner even faster than dehydration. Sabrina overcomes this by focusing on other runners, "taking out another headlamp," as she puts it. But for some, cannabis can return them to the present moment—the trees, the birds, the hypnotic rhythm of their own feet—long enough to push through some dark emotions.

There's a cruel irony to the fact that so many high-profile ultra-runners are secretly utilizing this "tool in your toolbox," as Meghan Hicks put it, while Avery, due to his branding himself as a stoner athlete, has to take extra precautions to never be caught with red eyes during a race.

After Avery landed first place in the Georgia Death Race (which landed him in the Western States 100, which, as you'll recall, is the biggest ultrarace in the nation), Boulder runner Dave Mackey took to social media to question the legitimacy of Avery's win, because he "is sponsored by companies that make PEDs," and says that he should've been drug-tested. (As of 2021, most ultraraces don't have the budgets for drug tests.)

The performance-enhancing drug in question was cannabis, a characterization that even Sabrina feels "blows things out of proportion." Though this debate rages on today throughout the trail-racing community.

"The biggest issue I had specifically with Avery," Mackey said on *The Dispatch Podcast*, "was that he's performing at an elite level and benefiting from [cannabis]. He's promoting the product and not being tested. If someone had been promoted by a steroid company, then I believe those people should be tested, especially once you are competing at a certain level, to make sure you are clean."

The dustup even inspired a comment on the issue from the American Trail Running Association (ATRA). "Whatever you're going to do that's legal, we're not going to judge," says Adam Chase, ATRA's president. "But having tried cannabis on a run, I can understand how it can be a performance enhancer. I'm glad it's a banned substance in competition."

After this incident, many races began drug-testing their top finishers, something unheard of in ultrarunning a few years earlier. Just to be extra cautious, Avery stops consuming weeks before a race and even volunteers to be drug-tested before approaching the starting line.

Despite her monumental success as a runner and the fact that she never touches cannabis, Sabrina has to be careful in how closely tied she is to her boyfriend when it comes to events and social media. As a runner, she's sponsored by several companies, the biggest being Altra shoes.* "Their founders were very Mormon and not the

---

* Since this interview, Sabrina has ended her relationship with Altra and is now sponsored by Adidas.

most open-minded people. After I won at Western States, I had law-yers and people from Altra reaching out to me, warning that I shouldn't be associated with any of Avery's marijuana stuff in any of my posts."

This is nothing new to Avery, who, despite gaining a lot of canna-bis sponsors, media attention, and fans for being the first profes-sional athlete to publicly declare his love of cannabis, has probably lost as many (if not more) fans and opportunities because of this.

"I got turned down by two shoe companies in the past couple months because of pot," he says. "Their US team managers were all on board for bringing me on the team, but when it made it to the international team, they shot it down so fast because they don't want anything to do with someone who's a cannabis advocate. It's bullshit, but it doesn't surprise me. I knew the moment I signed on the dotted line with my first marijuana sponsor I was crossing a bridge there was no turning back from. But I didn't care. I just wanted to cash my check and get back to running."

As we approach the end of the trail, I feel that I'm left with more questions than answers when it comes to competition and cannabis—and how the two play out in the young sport of ultrarun-ning. Neither Avery nor Sabrina strikes me as being like the psycho-logically toxic bullies I'd previously characterized all competitive athletes as. In fact, I have to confess a flutter of inspiration after having spent the afternoon with these two professional runners, and find myself wanting to plot a more ambitious course in my own running in the months ahead. I'm very curious about heart-rate training, heat exposure, and sprinting once a week in the hopes of increasing my speed and distance.

Is this a healthy mindset? I'm not sure, but I certainly feel a hun-ger for it.

When Steve Prefontaine's coach, Bill Bowerman, insisted he take a more calculated approach to his races, hanging back until the end and then rushing forward for the win, Pre balked at the idea (despite being an obsessively competitive runner), preferring a "pure guts race" and saying, "I don't want to win unless I know I've done my best, and the only way I know how to do that is to run out front, flat out until I have nothing left. Winning any other way is chickenshit."

The one thing I have learned for sure is that there is no singularly correct approach to running, just as there is no singularly correct approach to making art or taking drugs. Everyone I've spoken with is confident that ultrarunning—and the sporting world in general—will likely accommodate the role that cannabis can play in training and competition in the years ahead, and that will likely spark a lively debate about the true nature of this sport.

What we don't yet know will be the reasoning behind that shift: Will cannabis be viewed as a performance enhancer in competition, with all the intrigue and controversy that comes with that? Or will it be viewed as a tool of enlightenment, freeing athletes from the bonds of rivalry and centering them in the present moment of nature and the mind-body connection of physical activity?

Either way, this will potentially create a monumental sea change in sports. But it certainly won't be the first time. After all, it was only a few generations ago that Sabrina would have been forbidden to run more than two hundred meters in competition, lest her delicate female anatomy (as was believed by the male doctors at the time) collapse under the effort. Once we crossed that threshold, it quickly became ridiculous to see the issue any other way.

While myself and many others I've spoken with can attest to the physical and psychological wonders of cannabis as an exercise supplement, I'm beginning to realize that the naysayers aren't going to be swayed by any testimonials from a bunch of stoners. To further this conversation along, I am going to have to dig into the neuropharmacological science behind all this botanical mysticism.

What is going on in our brains and bodies when we consume cannabis? And what is it about that state that fits like a hand in a glove to the act of running?

Obviously, I won't be surprised when I learn that such a connection exists between the two. Though even someone as evangelical about the transcendent bliss of running high as myself will be shocked at just how fundamentally linked these two things are.

THE HAPPY CHEMICAL

WHAT IS THE NATURAL "RUNNER'S HIGH"? AND WHY DOES IT HAVE EVERYTHING TO DO WITH CANNABIS?

O, mickle is the powerful grace that lies
In herbs, plants, stones, and their true qualities.
For naught so vile that on the Earth doth live
But to the Earth some special good doth give.

—Friar Lawrence, *Romeo and Juliet*

RUN FOR YOUR LIFE

In the year 150,000 BC, a pack of humans are quietly stalking gazelles through the tall grass of the African savanna. They've been tracking their prey for three days now, and the humans are very tired and hungry. Someone's foot accidentally snaps a dry branch, and they're spotted, sending the herd sprinting away across the field. The humans take chase, but most of them give up quickly, as the gazelles are just too fast. One human continues though, and for storytelling purposes, we'll name him Gary.

Gary's bare feet slap the muddy ground, his naked body flailing in the sunshine as he sprints through the chest-high grass, no longer caring how much noise he's making. Gary has not eaten in a week. His body feels heavy, his tired muscles are cramping, and his joints are so swollen they radiate pain with each jostle of his sprinting legs. Though some part of Gary understands that if he fails to catch this animal, he will likely starve.

Narrowing his focus to one antelope, he chases her for so long, his friends see him disappear into the horizon. His lungs are burning, head dizzy, heart pounding so hard it can be seen through his skin. Just before Gary collapses in defeat under the blazing-hot sun, something amazing occurs.

The ache in his knees suddenly vanishes, as does the soreness in his feet. Gary's back straightens, head lifts, and stride lengthens. The gap between him and the antelope narrows as Gary begins to feel a bit lighter, each footstep suddenly a little easier. He's barely conscious of this, though. His entire being is absorbed in the chase, which comes to an end with five large steps and a screaming leap onto the antelope's back.

Fast-forward 152,000 years, and I'm running on a treadmill, fairly stoned, and reciting the Pledge of Allegiance. I am in the University of Colorado Boulder's Center for Innovation and Creativity, taking part in the groundbreaking study "Cannabis Use During Exercise." While I'm no fan of running on treadmills (they are to running what artificial insemination is to sex, I've always believed), I must admit that the gram of Tangerine Haze I just consumed has put me in quite a chipper mood, and my feet are springing along this moving side-walk with a graceful ease (reflected in my steady speech as I recite the pledge, which is how these scientists are testing my breathing during the study).

I'm here with Angela Bryan, the researcher behind the survey I mentioned earlier, who found that 80 percent of cannabis users in legalized states said that they got high before and/or after their workouts. A social and health psychologist who conducts research on health and risk behavior, Angela has spent the past two decades examining why we engage in unhealthy behavior and, perhaps more urgently, why we *do not* engage in healthy behavior—like exercise.

Why do so many people experience an emotional boost from ex-ercise, while the vast majority of the US population apparently does not?

According to the Centers for Disease Control, only 23 percent of Americans get a sufficient amount of exercise each week—which is defined as at least 150 minutes of moderate, or 75 minutes of vigor-ous exercise, in addition to muscle-strengthening activities at least twice a week. Setting aside our terrible diet and daily dose of stress, the sedentary issue alone costs the United States an extra $117 bil-lion in health-care expenses, the burden of which has led corporations to offer financial incentives to employees who track a sufficient number of steps on a Fitbit monitor. (I have a relative in Iowa with this arrangement, but he simply ties the Fitbit to his ankle and bounces his knee while sitting on the couch and updating his fantasy football teams.)

A whole galaxy of ailments inflicts those who do not move their bodies, most notably high blood pressure, heart disease, stroke, diabetes, and obesity. And there is an equally lengthy list of mental health detriments caused by inactivity—depression, anxiety, dementia, mood swings, and decreased acuity.

None of these sound very fun. In fact, they sound downright painful and scary.

So why are more than three-quarters of the people in the nation willing to endure such pain instead of taking a nightly walk in the park and doing a few push-ups each week? This was the riddle Angela Bryan had been trying to solve for years when she launched her survey asking people about their exercise habits.

"Your mental state is a huge factor when it comes to initiation and maintenance of exercise," Angela tells me. "In our work we often ask people how they feel when they're exercising. Is it enjoyable? Awful? Does it make you sad? And we find that people who are intrinsically motivated to exercise—they do it because they love it—they are more likely to keep doing it, and do it at a higher intensity. People who do it because their doctor or spouse told them to are less likely to maintain it."

Living and working in Boulder, Angela was stationed in ground zero of endurance-running culture—a scene made up of athletic psychopaths who just can't get enough exercise. It's an ideal buffet of fitness junkies for Angela to observe and contrast with the otherwise sedentary population of the rest of the country, ultimately raising the question: What made these people so different?

"Originally, our survey was not about cannabis and exercise," she says. "It was only one of several questions surrounding the possible risks and benefits of cannabis legalization and how it related to other health behaviors."

When the results showed that 80 percent of respondents in legalized states were using cannabis as part of their exercise regimen, Angela suddenly found herself spiraling down a cannabis-athletics rabbit hole, leading to myself and many others running on a treadmill in her lab under the influence of pot.

Could cannabis, Angela wondered, be the antidote to our sedentary lifestyle problem? Was there something about this plant that made people who loathe exercise suddenly enjoy it? And if so, what was the biomechanical dance between a human and this plant that could make such a thing possible?

To answer that question, we'll have to take a trip back to Israel in 1962, when a Bulgarian Holocaust survivor forever changed the game for cannabis science.

THE HAPPY CHEMICAL

Sporting a crew cut and tie, Raphael Mechoulam sits on a public bus with a pound of Lebanese hash on his lap. He's smiling brightly—still sporting the chubby cheeks of boyhood, despite years spent fleeing Nazis in the Bulgarian mountains—yet he's more than a little impatient as the Jerusalem traffic delays his trip from the police station to his chemistry lab.

Other bus patrons sniff the air, curious about the pungent aroma that recently entered the vehicle. It's definitely a . . . *different* smell, though no one clutches their pearls in disbelief. Mostly because no one on that bus has any clue what the scent is. While the popularity of cannabis has ebbed and flowed throughout history, by the early

1960s, drug laws have turned it into an underground novelty, both in Israel and in the States.

"Marijuana? Why would you want to study that? No one in the US smokes marijuana," a National Institutes of Health (NIH) representative told Raphael months earlier when he applied for a grant to research it. "Why don't you study something more relevant?"

As a Jewish immigrant who had narrowly escaped a trip to Auschwitz (his father wasn't so lucky), Raphael is eager to prove himself as a biochemical researcher. His homeland of Bulgaria had been torn between the growling jaws of Nazis and Soviets, leading to a carousel of propaganda spinning in unpredictable directions. Studying the tangible, consistent properties of the physical world gives him a sense of order. And he doesn't take that for granted.

Bored with developing insecticides for the Israeli army, Raphael is on the lookout for a topic obscure enough to be groundbreaking but relevant enough to score a grant from the United States. Multilingual and with a thirst for history, Raphael reads nineteenth-century medical texts from Russia, France, and Germany and keeps encountering a medicinal herb that, the texts claim, treats a seemingly endless list of ailments.

Cannabis.

Originating in central Asia, cannabis has been cultivated and consumed by humans as far back as 10,000 BC—basically since the birth of agriculture—while it's been growing on the planet for at least twenty-eight million years. Its uses as an industrial fiber could fill a book unto itself, but its role in Eastern medicine (with the West to follow centuries later) is equally profound.

The earliest texts of Chinese medicine, dating back to 2700 BC, list cannabis as a remedy for gout, malaria, constipation, menstrual cramps, and many other ailments. Ancient Egyptians used it for glaucoma and inflammation, as did the Greeks. The Hindus of India declared it "the food of the gods" (it does indeed contain a plethora of nutrients and protein when ingested) and used it to lower anxiety, overcome fatigue, enhance appetite, and aid sleep, among other benefits. The Zoroastrians of the Middle East listed it as the most important of all the ten thousand plant medicines in 700 BC, a sentiment shared by their Muslim successors centuries later. Recent archaeological evidence has also revealed THC-rich cannabis to be a part of Jewish rituals in ancient Israel, dating back 2,700 years.

Europeans eventually caught on in 1621, when medical texts declared it useful for depression, burns, irritable bowels, skin inflammation, coughs, jaundice, migraines, and much, much more.*

Cannabis elixirs were a common medicine throughout the first 150 years of American history (after all, early drafts of the Constitution were written on hemp paper, and the crop was treasured by many of our founding fathers), as were medical marijuana studies touting its vast number of benefits. Mary Todd ate hash for her anxiety after the death of her husband, Abraham Lincoln.

Cannabis had been a prominent medicine in the US pharmacopoeia for generations, yet Raphael found that research surrounding the plant had come to a near grinding halt a few decades into the twentieth century. With only a few exceptions, the herb that had been a staple of medicine throughout world history was suddenly absent from modern medical research. And it seems that will continue to be the case if Raphael can't get that NIH grant.

Despite prodigious use in the beatnik underground of Jack Kerouac and William Burroughs, few in mainstream America have heard of marijuana in 1962. (The Beatles are still two years away

....

* This brief sampling of medical marijuana throughout world history is woefully insufficient. To catalog all the ways this plant has been used by various cultures throughout the existence of humanity would require an *Infinite Jest*–level page count.

from their *Ed Sullivan Show* debut.) Luckily enough for Raphael, a US senator has just caught his son smoking pot, and he makes a call to the NIH asking what dangers await his child if this behavior continues. Forced to confront the fact that they have little to no modern research on the topic, someone at NIH mentions that a young Israeli scientist recently submitted a grant proposal to study cannabis.

And just like that, Raphael is in business.

"Luckily, we didn't have any legal trouble obtaining it," Raphael explains nearly a half century later, speaking to me via Skype from his home in Israel. "The police were very happy to give us hashish. Whenever we needed it, I would go and drink coffee with them, get five kilos, and take the bus to the lab. I doubt that would have been possible in many other places."

Considering how tricky it is for US researchers to get their hands on decent cannabis for research even today, it's hilarious how easily Raphael came across it in 1962. Looking back, it's an amazing set of fortuitous circumstances that allowed him to perform the most groundbreaking work in cannabis science to date—science that is now seen as revolutionary to his field, much as Albert Einstein's work is to engineering.

"It was strange to me that morphine and cocaine had been investigated thoroughly for many years," he says. "But with cannabis, which was in the same league of illicit drugs, the compounds [that affected humans] were still unknown."

Soon into his research on the police-provided hash, Raphael is able to isolate and map the structure of cannabis's main psychoactive ingredient, tetrahydrocannabinol, commonly known today as THC. In addition to delivering the euphoric intoxication pursued by recreational users, THC is also responsible for the anti-nausea and sedation effects (among others) of cannabis. Next, Raphael isolates and maps another compound, cannabidiol (CBD), which, it will later be discovered, can also deliver a number of health benefits—like treating schizophrenia and type 1 diabetes—without any of the intoxicating effects of THC. (Decades later, Republican senator Mitch McConnell will successfully push for THC-free hemp to be commercially manufactured in the United States, sparking an overnight boom in the CBD industry and promising relief from pain, anxiety, and insomnia.)

Raphael names these compounds "cannabinoids," and in the years to come more than 140 different types of them will be identified within the cannabis plant.

Despite decades of an increasingly antiscience, pro-incarceration war on drugs spreading across the Western world (making life for any US researcher investigating the therapeutic use of cannabis next to impossible), Raphael continues executing one groundbreaking study after another in the field of cannabis science over the next fifty years.

By the early eighties, he discovers the major elements of cannabis that interact with the human body and what the effects of that dance are—including a revolutionary study confirming what fifteenth-century Persians already knew: that CBD was profoundly effective at treating epileptic seizures. (The study would be ignored for thirty years.) Yet it was still not understood where in the brain and body these cannabinoids attach themselves.

Around this time, a US neuropharmacology researcher, Allyn Howlett, made an alarmingly curious discovery: instead of chaotically acting on a number of brain regions—the way amphetamines or other drugs do—cannabinoids seemed to fit like a lock and key into a set of cannabinoid receptors that resided in the brains of all mammals.

It appeared as if we were born to be high.

HIGH ON LIFE

The discovery of cannabinoid receptors inspired a question within Raphael that would revolutionize not only cannabis science but all of biological science: If we have cannabinoid receptors built into our brains, does that mean we manufacture our own internal cannabinoids?

It's not as farfetched as it might seem. After all, we have built-in opioid receptors that can be activated by derivatives of the poppy plant, like heroin or morphine, but function mainly to receive our own internal opioids like endorphins (a word that literally means "endogenous morphine"). It wouldn't be unprecedented for humans to have receptors for endogenous (internally manufactured) compounds that also happen to work as receptors for exogenous (outside the body) compounds.

By studying the activity of these cannabinoid receptors, Raphael and his team discover a neurotransmitter that seems to act upon our brains and bodies just as THC does. It is an endogenous cannabinoid. In addition to other functions, this cannabinoid appears to induce a pleasant euphoria in humans, as well as in all other vertebrate animals, providing a natural high that mirrors the neurological activity of someone who just smoked a joint.

Raphael is right: we do produce our own cannabis internally.

"Before we could publish [the findings], we had to give it a name," Raphael recalls. "We knew it had to do with positive moods, with happiness, and I wanted the word 'happiness' associated with it. There are a lot of languages spoken around Israel, but I couldn't find a word in French, English, or Hebrew that worked. There aren't a lot of words for 'happiness.'"

The principal author of this study, William Devane, has been learning the ancient Indian language of Sanskrit in his spare time and suggests to Raphael they use the word "ananda" in the naming of this endocannabinoid. In Hindu holy texts, "ananda" is the word for supreme happiness that follows a cycle of rebirth. And so they declare this joy-inducing neurotransmitter anandamide. (It was an appropriate reference considering the enormous role cannabis played in ancient Hindu cultures, which considered the plant "a gift to the world from the god Shiva," and featured it prominently in religious rites, medicine, and social life.)

Despite having little impact on marijuana laws or even modern medicine, the findings of Raphael's team revolutionize the study of mammalian biology. In the years ahead, his anandamide paper will be cited more than two thousand times by other researchers (practically unheard of in scientific circles) until the information becomes so well accepted there is no need to even reference the discovery—just as there is no need to cite Newton when researching gravity.

Soon it is established science that all vertebrate animals have an endocannabinoid system, which governs far more than just the herbal high of cannabis and the natural high of anandamide.

Beyond being just a mechanism of the brain, the receptors of the endocannabinoid system are found to be located throughout the body—in our skin, organs, bones, fat tissue, muscles, blood vessels, gastrointestinal tract—and the distribution of these cannabinoids regulates our systems of sleep, emotions, appetite, neuro-protection, pain, memory, immunity, reproduction, and much more. This profoundly complex, cell-signaling collection of enzymes, molecules, and receptors acts as a kind of matriarch of the entire body, making hundreds of micro-adjustments where needed to bring us back to a homeostasis of (ideal, if not perfect) health. Since this system plays a role in nearly every function of the body, its discovery provides an explanation for the mile-long list of ailments that medical marijuana is said to treat or cure.

Raphael will go on to become the rector of Hebrew University, honored around the world for his groundbreaking discoveries, and be regularly consulted on what cannabinoids—and what strains of cannabis—are appropriate for treating various illnesses. In 2013, the National Institutes of Health—the same US organization that once refused to fund Raphael, saying cannabis was "not relevant" to medical science—published a paper stating that "the endocannabinoid system is involved in essentially all human diseases."

Volumes of books could be written on the vast complexities of anandamide and the endocannabinoid system. Psychologically, physiologically, and even spiritually (if you're inclined to believe in such a thing) this network has a role to play in pretty much everything we as a species do, or is done to us. Though this is not a biology textbook. This is a book about the runner's high. Which makes what Raphael says to me at the end of our interview so wildly titillating.

"One of the reasons people exercise—whether they realize it or not—is to enhance the production of anandamide. You exercise, you feel better, and this is because of anandamide."

DID EVOLUTION "GIVE" US THE RUNNER'S HIGH?

While attending a fundamentalist Christian high school in rural Iowa, my science education mostly boiled down to this: God did it.

He built the world in seven days, and all of its mysterious beauty and complex interconnectivity exist within *His* master plan (and all suffering is due to the other guy). Ever since Evangelicals felt publicly humiliated in the 1927 Scopes Monkey Trial (when a Tennessee DA tried and failed to imprison an educator for teaching evolution, turning the redneck Christians into a freak show for the world's newspapers), the topic of evolution has been their white whale.

From then on, any discussion by Evangelicals surrounding the creation of the planet, or humans, would forever be couched within the framework of God's intentional hand, and was always contrasted against the absurd and shortsighted views of evolution—which cynically dismissed the awe-inspiring beauty of our world's mountains, rainstorms, laughing babies, bacon, and the music of Amy Grant as all just happening by anarchic chance.

This form of alt-science is known today as creationism, or "intelligent design." (It has a lot of cultural overlap with the flat-Earth movement.)

Conversely, evolutionary biologists have always been careful not to couch any mechanisms within us, or the planet—no matter how complex they may be interwoven—as being attributed to anything intentional. This doesn't mean they have no sense of awe for our world—Richard Dawkins's book *The Greatest Show on Earth* is basically a love letter to the overwhelming beauty of evolution—but such gratitude doesn't imply that a single, conscious entity deserves praise for this creation.

According to evolutionary biologists, it was through natural selection that we developed these bodies and the elaborate ecosystem they're dependent on—not as a result of an entity with a plan. In the early days of my science reporting I was often corrected on this point when interviewing evolutionary scientists and asking questions like, "When evolution gave us x, did it *intend* for us to become y?" and "Are we *designed* to be eating x, or did nature *want* us to be eating y?"

There's no "want" in nature, these scientists were quick to correct me. No "intend." No "design."

While I've shed my creationist roots and am fully on board with evolutionary science, I can't help but feel that romantic sense of design when looking at the natural reward systems built into our brains and bodies. Some of the most pleasurable aspects of being alive—food, sex, sleep, learning, and exercise—all happen to be the same activities that keep us alive. Isn't that crazy? Our post-pagan world view often teaches that pleasure (i.e., sin) leads to destruction, but—whether you attribute this to evolution or God—we are clearly hardwired to enjoy the things that are good for us.

Today we've hijacked some of these systems in unhealthy ways (and I'm speaking of processed foods here, not sex without procreation, which is common in nature). But the basic idea still rings true: Our desires teach us what we need—if we can learn to correctly listen to them, that is. The drive toward sex, sleep, and food is known as motivational salience, which means the desire is almost an instinctual reflex and does not need to be learned or consciously considered. The emotional rewards of exercise, however—particularly exercise with no obvious utility, like working out in a gym—require associative learning (i.e., you gotta experience it to believe it).

"There are multiple reward systems that act, from an evolutionary standpoint, to induce behavior," David Raichlen, professor of biological sciences at the University of Southern California, explains to me. "The two major reward systems are endocannabinoids and endorphins. Both of them are powerful pain relievers, and so when it comes to exercise, there's a reward of pain relief, allowing you to move longer distances, consume more calories, survive longer, and pass on your genes. When these pathways enter the brain, there's a mental health reward—a good feeling."

With an olive-skinned, southern European handsomeness, David resembles a slimmer version of *Mad Men*'s Jon Hamm. A lifelong runner and science geek, he's always been fascinated by the evolutionary mechanisms influencing our physical proclivity for running—and why it makes us feel so damn good.

David is perhaps best known for his work with paleontologist

Daniel Liebman, featured in the book that inspired the barefoot running craze, *Born to Run*. Throughout a set of experiments, David and Daniel revealed that despite previously accepted wisdom, humans were the ultimate distance runners of the animal kingdom. We may not be able to sprint as fast as a cheetah or a horse, but due to a number of physical traits—sweat glands, springy Achilles tendons, wide shoulders, muscular butts (that also act as a kind of tail)—we have the ability to outrun any animal over long distances.

We're the steady tortoise that outlasts the speedy hare.

There is substantial paleontological evidence that we evolved this ability somewhere around two million years ago as a method of hunting gazelles across the African savanna. As humans, we're not the fiercest creatures; our mouths and hands don't make for the most terrifying weapons. So even if we could chase down our prey over short distances, we'd have a much harder time subduing them than a tiger or wolf might. Though it seems that, across the globe, humans learned that if they tracked their prey long enough (particularly on hot days), running no faster than a ten-minute mile, they could wear the animal down into a state of paralytic heat stroke.

And then, voilà, a rock or a spear could easily finish the job.

It wasn't the most valiant hunting method, but it proved reliable, keeping our species alive long enough for us to evolve a set of physical features that made the job even easier. Today, whenever the millions of marathon runners across the world run their 26.2 miles, they're actually reenacting an ancient hunting ritual of wearing down game with steady persistence—a ritual they owe their articulate feet, meaty calves, and swinging arms to.

Whether by design or natural selection, we are clearly born to run—at least physically. Though following these studies, David wondered if there was more to this system than just the ideal set of legs. After all, scores of people all over the world continue to run every day, and very few of them are chasing down their dinner.

They're chasing that mythical, psychotropic shift known as the "runner's high."

The term had been thrown around a lot ever since the running boom of the 1970s and '80s, but there was very little science surrounding it. Mostly because it was a subjective, private experience, reliant on the anecdotal descriptions of sweaty, smiling runners at the end of a long jog. A lot of runners claim that they've never experienced such a thing, or only felt it once or twice—though from a scientific standpoint, it's a very difficult thing to define.

Whatever it was, David wondered if the sensations described by those experiencing a runner's high—euphoria, decreased anxiety, increased appreciation of nature, shifting perception of time—could be part of some evolutionary reward system that would aid us in our endurance hunting. Perhaps we weren't born to be just *good* at running but also born to *enjoy* running.

But how could you possibly document and study such emotional states?

A 2003 study published in the *British Journal of Sports Medicine* revealed that when athletes ran at around 70 percent of their maximum heart rate for fifty minutes, the levels of anandamide in their blood rose dramatically. Familiar with Raphael Mechoulam's discoveries surrounding this endocannabinoid named for the state of bliss, researchers began to wonder whether anandamide was playing a role in the so-called runner's high. A later study on mice revealed that when their endocannabinoid receptors were removed, the mice suddenly no longer found any joy in running on their treadmill, and they stopped doing it.

These studies were part of a growing tide of research surrounding anandamide and the endocannabinoid system after Raphael Mechoulam's discoveries in the 1990s. Suddenly researchers with no previous interest in cannabis were finding themselves investigating the same neurobiological systems activated by millions of Deadheads around the world. Due to the stigma surrounding cannabis (which was taboo enough to kill funding and even careers in the US science world), many endocannabinoid-system researchers declined to acknowledge this system's botanical cousin in their research. While others found themselves newly curious about medical marijuana, discovered the wealth of historical research on the subject—as well as the modern silencing of it—and became advocates for more cannabis research.

CANINES AND CANNABIS

Before my journalism career took off, I spent a few years as a dog walker.

This was long before I started running, back when my soft, listless body worked overtime to process all the booze and nicotine in my system. I was a poor match for the dogs' primal puppy energy, so I would take them to a nearby park with my skateboard, allowing them to crank it up to 11 while I just rolled along, letting my wheels do the work. They didn't want to go anywhere specific—they just wanted to *go*!

I'd crouch down low, sandwiched between a pair of Australian shepherds or Rhodesian ridgebacks galloping at full speed. There, moving with the pack, I'd see a wild, feverish joy spread across their faces. Eyes wide and dilated, mouths open in goofy grins, tongues lolling, limbs pumping with urgent rhythm—it was a look I recognized from years of attending raves and rock festivals.

These dogs were getting high from running.

I saw this all the more when I got my first puppy, a sprightly German short-hair-pointer mix I named Iggy (after the most athletic rock performer in history, Iggy Pop). No amount of walks could satisfy the turbine spinning within him, so I'd take Iggy to the park so that he could wear himself out with the other dogs while I smoked cigarettes. The second I'd unhook him, Iggy would transform into a sprinting machine, legs churning so fast they'd blur like the pistons of a cartoon locomotive. He would taunt every dog in the park into chasing him, and once he had a dozen of them on his tail, I'd see this look come over him: mouth open, eyes growing large and feverish, like the face of a skydiving Jack Nicholson.

"Dogs will run even when they are not hungry, and they derive pleasure from the hunt itself," writes biologist Bernd Heinrich in *Why We Run.* "Dogs will gladly retrieve such symbolic prey as sticks and Frisbees. The pleasure they get from these activities is, as running is with us, partly social. . . . Cats are not socially motivated like dogs or humans. No matter how many times you make a cat run around a track, it will not race."

At the time, I had no idea these dogs were (unconsciously) tapping into the same evolutionary reward systems that I would eventually embrace years later when I got a taste for the runner's high. And I certainly never could've predicted it was all linked to cannabis.

But that was just what David Raichlen was pondering when he arranged for some dogs, ferrets, and humans to run on a treadmill in his lab.

After working with Daniel Liebman on his *Born to Run* studies and encountering research that revealed running led to an increase in anandamide levels in humans, David wanted to investigate whether the endocannabinoid system was a key player (if not the central operator) in the runner's high. Thankfully, there happened to be a rising star in the field working just down the hall at the University of Arizona, where David was working at the time.

With the exception of a joint he'd tried at a Def Leppard concert back in 1988, Greg Gerdeman had little interest in cannabis while pursuing a career in neuroscience. After becoming obsessed with the theory of "retrograde messengers"—essentially neurotransmitters flowing in the opposite direction they're wired to—and publishing groundbreaking work that showed anandamide was behaving just this way, he became a kind of wunderkind in the emerging field of endocannabinoid science—the equivalent of being a computer coding expert in the 1980s.

"I read every endocannabinoid paper that came out, which at first was only a handful of papers worldwide [in 1996]. There was still a lot of stigma around the subject," Greg recalls decades later. Trim and healthy, with a baseball cap and a bit of scruff, his appearance looks basic enough that he doesn't stand out as a scientist, yet loose enough that he fits in with the counterculture world of marijuana. "In time there were a handful of endocannabinoid papers coming out each week. Now there are hundreds of them every month. It's become one of the most epic advances in physiological science in the last fifty years."

For Greg, it was impossible to ignore the role of cannabis in studying the endocannabinoid system. In time he found himself straddling the culturally disparate worlds of mainstream science and the burgeoning medical marijuana scene of California (which became the first state to legalize medical marijuana, in 1996).

Soon Greg was writing for cannabis publications like *O'Shaughnessy's* (under a pseudonym, for fear of risking his access to grant funding) and spending time with underground marijuana growers. Witnessing the aggressive raids by the DEA of these simple hippie pot farmers—often involving vandalism, automatic weapons, violent arrests, costly court appearances, and sometimes death, despite cannabis being legal at the state level—Greg found himself firmly on one side of the ideological line. "I became convinced that these people are saints, they're helping sick people, and the feds are unnecessarily terrorizing them."

Around 2007, David Raichlen knocked on Greg's office door at the University of Arizona, asking if he'd be interested in working on a study on whether endocannabinoids are a part of an evolutionary reward system for running. The idea intrigued him, as he'd had several friends in college who were part of a running group that got high before long runs, and he knew that anandamide acted almost exactly like THC on the brain and body. So it stood to reason that anandamide could be the source of the runner's high.

"Greg was one of the few people who was an expert in endocannabinoids, which was not my area of expertise," recalls David. "I needed someone with neuroscience and pharmacological expertise, while I had an evolutionary and comparative biology perspective. With questions like this, you need to converge different disciplines."

But if all vertebrate animals had an endocannabinoid system, and anandamide performed an endless number of jobs in our brains and bodies, how would you determine if it's part of the evolutionary running reward system?

"We looked at animals with different evolutionary histories of endurance running," says David. "Some were natural runners, like dogs and humans, while others were not, like ferrets. And for ethical reasons we didn't want to use animals that would be harmed or euthanized, so we used pet dogs and adopted out the ferrets at the end of the study."

It would've been fascinating to include chimps in the study, as they share 98 percent of our DNA yet never run more than a few yards, but both researchers were very concerned about animal safety and wanted to study only those species that could be safely obtained and adopted after the study.

Predictably, the athletic humans and happy-go-lucky dogs had a fine time running on the treadmill, while the ferrets—which typically sleep thirteen hours each night, and almost never run more than a few yards in a day—were less enthusiastic. At least this would appear to be the case in their bloodwork. After running for thirty minutes at 70 percent heart rate, the humans and dogs had major increases in anandamide, compared with blood taken before the workout, while the ferrets did not.

When Greg and David explain these results to me, I think of the smiling face of my dog, Iggy, as well as the huskies I used to skate alongside in Denver parks, an obvious surge of joy coursing through their veins whenever they would engage in a run.*

"Like a lot of human societies, dogs, when hunting, will often exhaust their prey," says Greg. "African hunting dogs will chase a gazelle for miles and miles until they just drop."

Just like humans, dogs evolved a runner's high for survival. And also just like us, while living a life of convenience and comfort, they continue to push that button just for the hell of it, because it feels so damn good to cut loose and run through a grassy park (or, in Iggy's case, to taunt other dogs into racing him).

The differing test results between the dogs and humans, on the one hand, and the ferrets, on the other, suggests that "maybe this is not just a ubiquitous mechanism across all animals," David wondered, "but there's something specific about your evolutionary history that links faster movement to the endocannabinoid system."

But not *too* fast.

When taken above 70 percent maximum heart-rate threshold—into a commanding sprint—human participants did not experience increased anandamide levels. Nor did the participants walking at a gentle pace on the treadmill (though other studies have shown small anandamide increases with walking). The pace that delivered the

---

* In case you were wondering, there are a number of medical marijuana applications for dogs—who have the same endocannabinoid system that we do. There are both psychoactive and nonpsychoactive cannabis products given to pets with pain, anxiety, and epilepsy. News reports on this have been a source of great humor for conservative, anti-pot commentators.

highest spikes in these joy-inducing neurotransmitters was a comfortable jog of around a ten-minute mile. The same pace that endurance hunters are believed to have jogged at throughout history.

"I've been out with foragers in Tanzania, and they don't go very fast," says David. "Your heart rate is up, but it's still a nice moderate to moderate-intense pace that you can do for hours."

The study also included a psychological evaluation of each of the human runners, measuring the emotional effect of the experience. "The increase in feelings of well-being with each of these runners and the amount of anandamide in their bloodstream was very tightly correlated," recalls Greg. "It was much closer than I'd expected, which really blew me away."

"MY ENDORPHINS ARE KICKING IN!"

So if an increase in anandamide is responsible for the runner's high, where does that leave endorphins? After all, the word "endorphin" is practically synonymous with "post-workout euphoria." A casual Google search of the word brings up articles from Wikipedia and WebMD ascribing the emotional benefits of exercise to endorphins (it also brings up a fitness center two miles from my house named Endorphins).

Seeing as anandamide is an endogenous cannabinoid and endorphins are an endogenous opioid, a crude way to phrase this debate would be, Is it our internal heroin or weed that causes the runner's high?

Around the same time that David was observing humans on a treadmill, Johannes Fuss was conducting similar experiments across the pond at the University of Hamburg, Germany. Though he wasn't examining dogs or ferrets, he was looking at the endorphin activity of humans and mice engaged in exercise, convinced of the same thing that David Raichlen was learning: it was likely that anandamide, not endorphins, was the source of the runner's high.

"The idea that endorphins cause the runner's high is one of the few things that generated from popular belief but is still connected to science," Johannes explains to me. Speaking in a thick German accent, Johannes resembles a young David Beckham with his wide smile, tightly cropped beard, and buzzcut. "People who are exercising will say, 'My endorphins are kicking in!' as it's a very popular phrase. But there was no proof of this."

The "endorphins" explanation never sat well with Johannes.

He was seeing an increasing amount of research around anandamide and exercise and wanted to put the endorphin theory to the test. Throughout a series of studies, Johannes duplicated research showing an increase in anandamide in mice running on wheels, as well as in humans on treadmills, but also, most interestingly, found no change in the behavior of mice running on wheels whose opioid receptors (which process endorphins) were blocked.

"We repeated that experiment with sixty [human] endurance runners on treadmills, half of whom were given opioid blockers and the other a placebo, and a comparable number of people in both groups had the runner's high of increased euphoria and reduced anxiety. There is even evidence showing that opioid blockage does not prevent the reduction of pain during exercise in humans. So I'm pretty skeptical that opioids play a role in the runner's high."

WHAT DOES "HIGH" EVEN MEAN?

While his research depended on asking participants if they were experiencing a "runner's high," Johannes admits that there isn't always a universally understood definition of this sensation, and this sometimes complicates the self-reporting aspect of these experiments.

"Some people say they have it every time, others say they've never had it, but it really depends on how you define it," says Johannes. "People don't think of the same thing when they say 'runner's high.' When asked, only thirty percent of participants in our study said they felt the runner's high, but they all reported feelings of euphoria."

David Raichlen says that the runner's high—in some form—is universal.

"Most of the psychology work done on this shows there aren't groups of people who don't feel better after they exercise," he says. "They may not recognize it right away, or they don't link those two things, but if they exercise correctly, it's there. For some there may also be a kind of fitness hump they need to get over. There's a correlation between intensity and anandamide release—really high or really low intensity doesn't do it—so one hypothesis could be that people who are new to exercise may have a hard time staying in that moderate intensity. They're either going really slow, or they overshoot and go into that high-intensity zone. It may take time before you have the cardiovascular system required to stay in that moderate zone for twenty to thirty minutes."

"I prefer to call it the 'runner's joy' instead of the 'runner's high,'" says Greg Gerdeman, since some people negatively associate the word "high" with countercultural tropes of laziness and intoxication.

Johannes also notes that contextual factors like music and setting are big influencers on mood when running, making it difficult to nail down a single culprit. "When asking subjects if they've felt a runner's high before, some will say, 'Yeah, often when I'm listening to this certain song, and running in this landscape and thinking of my partner, I'll have a runner's high.' It's not just the body releasing hormones. It's also the context."

For some, it's not just the waves of euphoria that define the runner's high but a reprieve from the pain, anxiety, and stubborn lethargy that typically plague any attempt at physical movement. As David Raichlen noted, some poor souls might not be able to summit the cardio threshold required to reach the natural runner's high and may require a little botanical push to get there.

CHRONIC RELIEF

Naturally, a lot of people in the fitness community are skeptical of the benefits of cannabis. After decades of propaganda falsely claiming that cannabis users are lazy and unhealthy, while athletes are championed as sober, dedicated souls of grit and respectability, there's a lot of drama in this culture clash. Opponents often ask for more definitive science, but the obstacles researchers must navigate to explore this topic are, at the moment, insurmountable.

We'll explore this deeper in chapter five, but it basically boils down to this: studies about the benefits of cannabis often don't get funding or approval from government and academic agencies.

When Jonathan Lisano conducted his study on athletes who get high, at the School of Sport and Exercise Science at the University of Northern Colorado, it had to first be framed as an examination of how cannabis *negatively* impacted exercise. This is the dark irony of nearly all cannabis research in the United States: any revelation of its charms must be couched in a study of its harms.

After years of anecdotal reports of professional athletes using cannabis (or those who formerly hated exercise suddenly embracing it thanks to edibles), Jonathan was eager to pioneer this popular yet under-researched fitness trend. However, many at UNC feared their reputation could be in jeopardy for being the first to marry themselves to the idea that weed made you good at sports.

"It took a lot longer to get approval for our studies than it would any other," Jonathan explains to me. "We had to be careful in the language we used to describe the aims of our research, phrasing it to sound neutral, or to even suggest that we were looking for the potential harms of cannabis to young athletes."

Along with Dr. Laura Stewart, he was eventually able to develop a cannabis research lab (with the intention of exploring the intersection of cannabis and athletics) but wasn't allowed to bring any cannabis onto the campus, administer it to any participants, or explore any overtly positive aspects of the plant.

However, he was able to conduct surveys that explored the variety of ways athletes used cannabis, and compare that with the research we already have on the plant's impact on humans and animals. He was also able to study the athletic performance of these stoners in the lab itself.

Those who regularly consumed cannabis were matched on a treadmill against those who never used—accounting for age, health, and fitness level—and the results revealed no difference between the two groups in regard to body composition, VO_2 max, performance, or cortisol levels. A later survey of his revealed that 92 percent of cannabis athletes got high before their workout began, 60 percent said they used no particular strain, and all of them said they used it for pain relief—among many other reasons.

In addition to anxiety, boredom, and lethargy, relief from pain is both a central feature of the natural runner's high and a selling point for the CBD craze that has swept the nation. Particularly with seniors looking to become more active.

Lia Oriel* teaches a cannabis fitness class in Boulder and says

....

* Lia was also one of the participants in Jonathan's cannabis athletes study, which was where she learned she had an exceptionally high VO_2 max, allowing her to casually jump into marathons with little to no training. Known to her friends as "the Hummingbird," she'll appear again in a later chapter.

that seniors make up a large percentage of her clients—who often appreciate her willingness to visit a dispensary on their behalf. "Most of them had never used marijuana before and were intimidated by dispensaries," she tells me. "A lot of them like the THC sublingual sprays, and the CBD lotion for their joints. One elderly couple I set up with stationary bikes on their porch and some chocolate edibles, and she's never felt such relief in her knees, and he got off trazodone for sleeping, which is huge."

Among the vast catalog of medical marijuana use throughout world history, seeking relief from the mental and bodily pains of physical activity is well documented. European travelers to India in the sixteenth century noted that many field laborers used hemp prodigiously throughout the day. A similar observation was made years later of fishermen in Jamaica, who, studies show, have improved night vision when consuming THC, as well as Jamaican laborers of all stripes, who reportedly cite an increase in energy and a lift in spirit when performing mundane, tedious labor.

Zulu warriors would consume cannabis (either via smoke, enema, or steam bath) to rouse their courage before battle, a dynamic that translates to the psychological hurdles facing modern-day athletes.

Many athletes say that cannabis reduces their anxiety enough to overcome the fear of daredevil activities—like the parachuting skiers Roger Boyd met in France. It also allows athletes to overcome the anxiety of returning to their sport after an injury, which is cited by the World Anti-Doping Agency (WADA) as one of the reasons the substance is banned in competition.

A great deal of effort has been put into retroactively proving that cannabis makes a person lazy, while unintentionally showing the opposite.

A 2016 study on rats exposed to moderate doses of THC revealed its energizing, antianxiety effects, creating a desire to run and play more than usual in the rodents. Though this same study also revealed the biphasic effect of cannabis, showing that in excessive doses the opposite impact (lethargy, anxiety) can also set in. Similar to the runner's high requiring a wholesome trot (not a walk, not a sprint) for around thirty minutes before the euphoria-inducing anandamide surge kicks in, the desired effect of cannabis use during exercise is also very dose-dependent.

Though if we have cannabinoids naturally flowing within us, why do we need to consume cannabis? Well, considering that only 5 percent of the US population exercises each day (and a certain amount of even that number probably hate it), logic would suggest that a great deal of people have difficulty achieving exercise-induced euphoria. Some of this is likely due to David Raichlen's theory that many people new to exercise either go too hard too fast or go wildly slow, and it takes some time to comfortably enter that sweet spot of 70 percent heart rate for the required thirty minutes to feel that jolt of anandamide.

Though for some, even the perfect amount of cardio can fail to induce the runner's high. This is possibly due to a medical condition known as clinical endocannabinoid deficiency, which results in misfires of the endocannabinoid system, often resulting in irritable bowel syndrome, fibromyalgia, and migraines. Ultimately, any use of cannabis is an alteration of the endocannabinoid system one way or another, but CED is a more severe condition resulting from either genetics or lifestyle.

Neurologist, former senior medical adviser to GW Pharmaceuticals, and cannabis science icon, Dr. Ethan Russo first coined the term "CED" in a 2001 research paper. (We'll be hearing from Ethan a lot in this book, as he graciously becomes the trusted expert I call at all hours to satisfy my random cannabis curiosities.) Years before he'd theorized that if an illness such as Parkinson's was due to misfiring dopamine, as clinical depression was with serotonin, it stood to reason that an even more important neurotransmitter like anandamide would be subject to misfiring and lead to a whole catalog of ailments. Several follow-up studies proved this to be true.

"The endocannabinoid system is extremely complex, and to break down how cannabis impacts it would take hours," Ethan explains to me over the phone one night. "But one thing we do know is that THC and CBD, in small amounts, will jump-start this system and increase anandamide release."

This would explain the common story I hear so often from pothead runners: cannabis delivers the runner's high quicker. So for those who have difficulty experiencing it, cannabis could be a possible ticket into the bliss of running.

And if they enjoy it, they're much more likely to keep doing it.

Or at least this was Angela Bryan's theory when she encouraged me to smoke pot and run on a treadmill in her lab. Does cannabis make exercise more fun? For myself and so many others, this does seem to be the case. But is this due to cannabinoid misfires being corrected by an herbal supplement, or does pot offer an additional therapeutic benefit beyond just neurotransmitters and anti-inflammatories?

For many, the cultural associations with exercise—often revolving around male dominance, the toxic shame of diet culture, and the existential anxiety of dying young without it—are so powerful they keep many of us from taking that first step into an evening walk around the neighborhood. Does cannabis have the power to change this?

In the weeks ahead, I'll meet a combat veteran, a wheelchair athlete, and a formerly incapacitated single mother who will reveal just how fundamentally transformative cannabis has the power to be. For both the body *and* the mind.

LET'S FORGET PHYSICAL

HOW CANNABIS CHANGES
THE WAY WE RELATE TO EXERCISE

> We are all in the gutter, but some of us
> are looking at the stars.
>
> —Oscar Wilde

UNCONSCIOUS CARDIO

When I said I'd hated exercise before cannabis, that was a lie.

From the days in my mother's womb to around the age of eighteen, I engaged in some form of Pentecostal worship at least once or twice a week. For those who haven't seen documentaries like *Jesus Camp* or *Marjoe*, a Pentecostal church service involves intense shaking, sprinting, jumping up and down, speaking in tongues (i.e., holy gibberish), and dramatically collapsing to the floor when touched by the pastor. It was a primal, sweaty ritual that would sound like an orgy of feral cats were a recording of it played to the untrained ear.

While I was chubby and sedentary the rest of the time (looking not unlike Bobby from *King of the Hill*), I loved the feeling of pushing my body to the extreme, feeling my heart pound and lungs burn. At the time, I attributed this euphoria to a blessing from the Holy Spirit, though today I would view it as an influx of cardio-induced anandamide.

Whatever it was, I certainly never called it "exercise."

Years later—after my faith abandoned me—I tapped into these same neural networks at dance clubs. Every Friday in Denver an event called Lipgloss spun all my favorite music (indie rock, Brit pop, eighties hits, glam-rock). My personal devotion to these songs and the sentiments behind them equaled my teenage zeal for Jesus. The music would drive me to Iggy Pop levels of flailing, stomping, spinning, and head-snapping aerobics. Considering how out of shape—and drunk—I was at the time, it wouldn't take long for me to reach my max heart rate and become so light-headed I'd need to collapse on the nearest shoulder.

Eventually, this ritual became unsustainable for a number of reasons.

Looking back now, after several years of running high, I can see that my routine of cannabis, loud music, and hours of cardio has been an unconscious attempt to recapture those Pentecostal teens and heady twenties on the dance floor. I'm much happier now as a stoned runner, but I can't help but note how much more pure, honest, and natural this behavior was when I didn't think of it as exercise. I never thought of it as anything other than a playful good time.

Never in the church or the dance club was I motivated to burn excess calories, strengthen my cardiovascular system, or improve my neural health (even if those were the unintended benefits). I was just rocking out. And that's a difficult state to achieve with our modern understanding of the term "exercise."

When I first met the Man Who Runs with Goats, I'd been training for my first ultramarathon and was kind of hating it. Feeling insecure about writing a book on ultraraces while never tackling one myself, I buckled down into a disciplined routine of sprints, splits, slow runs, long runs, strength training, and endless hours of stretching late into the night and early morning.

I wasn't feeling competitive with Avery and Sabrina, but I was inspired to run at their level. Even if that wasn't possible, it was where I'd set my sights. I wanted to casually scale a mountain like a leaping antelope, run for days and nights at a time like the Tarahumara runners of Mexico. I wanted a strong body that was ready for whatever a mountain could throw at me.

I got into heart-rate training, nose breathing, paleo eating, and intermittent fasting. I bought a heart-rate monitor, posture corrector, IT-band strap, massage gun, muscle scraper, foot roller, athletic bath-bombs, and a whole galaxy of different running shoes (from maximal to minimal, from custom-made orthotics to "barefoot" shoes).

In the end, I was pushing my body so hard that my performance actually declined—and I began to view running the way most Americans do: as a miserable obligation. Lost was the goofy weirdness of Pentecostalism, the kinetic gyrations of the dance floor, and all that was left was the cold reality of another lap around the park.

This is the ultimate conundrum anyone with ambitions for greatness encounters. You get excited about a lofty goal, but in your myopic pursuit of something out of your reach, you lose touch with the present. You lose sight of the childlike wonder that made the thing appealing in the first place. This is what Avery Collins was getting at when he spoke of the balance between focusing on the numbers and maintaining your joy.

Thankfully, we live in the age of legal weed (or at least I do in Colorado), providing an escape hatch from the neurotic misery of our minds, a way to abandon the depression of the past and the anxiety of the future and to settle into the gorgeous, playful present.

THE MAN WHO RUNS WITH GOATS

I have to admit, this is not how I pictured an earthship.

When Brent Connell told me over the phone about his house made of 100 percent recycled materials that generates its own energy and operates in biological harmony with the ecosystem around it, I imagined something a bit more jumbled and rudimentary, like the scores of homeless encampments in Denver, made of randomly procured objects. But instead I find a charming horizontal structure framed in beige stucco, almost cartoonish in its elegant minimalism, reminding me a bit of the homes in *The Flintstones* movie.

Most of it appears as just one long wall of glass resting on a grassy hill.

The majority of it is situated beneath the ground.

When I heard about all the chickens, dogs, cats, goats, llamas, alpacas, deer, and bees that shared this property—none for agricultural purposes—I pictured a chaotic Doctor Dolittle world. But the acreage is empty and peaceful when I come down the driveway, and it'll be hours before all the animals introduce themselves. Brent Connell—the Man Who Runs with Goats—isn't what I expected either.

A three-legged Doberman hops alongside him as he approaches my car, a stocky lumberjack of a man with a biker beard and sleeves of tattoos. His gruff face and hulking demeanor make me think of the Denver club bouncers I never wanted to find myself on the wrong side of. But when he leans into my window, removes his sunglasses, and introduces himself, I'm struck by a pair of the gentlest, most vulnerable blue eyes I've ever seen.

I've traveled to a rural piece of property outside Colorado Springs to meet this man, who, as a friend explained to me, likes to get high and run with animals.

Over the last few years, whenever anyone hears that I like to get stoned and run, they often say, Oh weird, I have a friend/sister/boss/ whatever who does the same thing, but I didn't think anyone else did. This was the case when I was told about Brent Connell via his brother, and my curiosity was tickled enough to make the trip for a few reasons: (1) I'm fascinated by running with pack animals; (2) Brent grows his own cannabis, and therefore has ultimate control over the nuances of his product; and (3) he lives in an earthship, a fascinating architectural trend that efficiently harnesses natural resources for low-cost, off-the-grid energy, which allows him to spend nearly all his time isolated in the Rocky Mountains.

He's also a combat veteran who successfully treated his severe PTSD by running high in nature. But I don't know that yet.

Brent invites me inside the earthship, which is very long and slim, designed to absorb as much sunshine as possible through its entirely glass south-facing wall. My body sighs pleasantly, breathing in air oxygenated by hundreds of plants, gently humidified by trickling fountains and an elaborate irrigation system. The floor is stone tile, with skylights illuminating every room. A bed of flowers, vegetables, herbs, cacti, and cannabis plants rests beneath the glass wall. The wall is perfectly angled to let in warm sunlight during the winter and reflect it during the summer.

"It'll be five degrees outside in the middle of winter, but we're walking around in here in our underwear," says Courtney Connell, Brent's wife. "I miss Chinese and pizza delivery, being so far out here, but it's definitely worth it."

It's remarkably cozy, the kind of place you'd like to spend the weekend during a blizzard, curled up with a good novel and endless cups of tea. Or an ideal place to nurse the psychological wounds of war.

At one point Brent looks over my shoulder and says, "Here comes trouble."

I turn to look out through the 150-foot-long glass wall and gasp.

Emerging from an afternoon fog are around thirty baby deer, clumsily walking toward the earthship. My twee little heart melts as we all walk outside, the excited Doberman playing in the grass as Courtney feeds the baby deer. "This one was born in a hailstorm, then got lost and separated from his mother," Courtney tells me. "Then he ran into a stable, where he was kicked in the head by a horse, giving him brain damage."

What a cruel introduction to life, I think.

I'm told these deer are part of an adjacent animal refuge that both Courtney and Brent volunteer with. When I learn that the rest of Brent's time is spent doing handiwork for the half-dozen retired widows that live nearby, along with an old man with Parkinson's, I'm beginning to pick up on a theme.

It's like the Island of Misfit Toys: Wildlife Edition.

Though Brent doesn't speak much; and so this whole caring-for-broken-things vibe I'm getting is never overtly stated (not even as a humblebrag). In fact, Brent's life transitioned from PTSD-stricken vet living a life of panic in the city to this mountain sanctuary of weed, trail running, and soft-eyed baby deer so gradually he often forgets the deliberate decisions that brought him here in the first place. Most of the time, life here is so good he'd rather not think about life before the earthship (though for trauma survivors, re-membering isn't always voluntary).

"When Brent came back from Iraq, he was very different, and he couldn't handle life in the city," Courtney tells me, sitting on a patio chair while petting a cat on her lap. "Neither of us knew what was going on. We were both broke and in school, so there was a lot of stress anyway. We never even thought of PTSD. But he never wanted to go out dancing or be social like he used to. He'd have night terrors and wake up covered in sweat. He couldn't handle being in restau-rants with his back exposed, and he'd fly into a rage over the littlest thing, hate himself for it, then pull away from me. . . . He's never told me everything that happened to him over there, but I've put a few pieces together. I know that he saw body parts, I know vehicles were blown up with people inside. But I don't know who those peo-ple were in relation to him."

I look up and see Brent, smiling and walking toward us as two adolescent goats come bounding past him down the grassy hill, oc-casionally springing their heels off to one side like skateboarders.

"I never felt in danger of him," Courtney continues, and I look back to her. "He was never violent. He would get his rage out on the runs. Actually, the cannabis was first, and that helped him let his guard down and relax, because over there he could never relax. You're always on alert. Everyone potentially has a bomb: the children, the donkeys, the women, the old men. And he couldn't turn that off when he came home. Running ultramarathons gave him the time and space to sort things out."

Admittedly, I'm having a difficult time paying attention. As Courtney is talking, two Nigerian dwarf goats are fighting over who gets to eat my shoelaces.

"They're ten-month-old brothers, so they're nearly grown but are still a bit spastic," Brent tells me. "The white one is Frisco, the brown one is Breckenridge. They're just pets, really. We take them backpacking with us. And running. You wanna run?"

I do indeed.

We share a quick joint (Courtney declines, as she imbibes only on special occasions), Brent straps on a pair of Luna sandals, and soon we're off, jogging down a dirt road with two young goats and a three-legged dog named Remyington.

"So were you always into running?" I ask, trying to keep my breath steady as he guides us onto the half-marathon trail that circles his property.

"No way," he says. "For most of my life I hated running. Throughout my eight years in the Air Force I hated it so much I could barely handle the two-mile PT test. Cannabis had a lot to do with changing that."

Like myself, Brent grew up in a conservative Christian family, where his father was the pastor of a Pentecostal church. He rebelled much earlier than I did though, immersing himself in the heavy metal world that inspired the Satanic Panic of the 1990s. After a bull-riding phase in high school, the military was a natural course for Brent and his friends, as the largest Air Force academy in the world was just a few miles away.

Courtney and Brent married shortly before Brent was shipped off to Iraq in 2004, and whatever happened in the six months he was there, it was enough to fundamentally change his personality when he came home. Naturally, if Brent has a difficult time discussing this with his wife, he's not likely to open up about it to a journalist he just met, though small details emerge in our conversation. I learn he had multiple jobs in Iraq, working as both a prison guard and a mechanic. When explaining how he injured his back changing a truck tire too quickly, Brent seasons the story with an ominous detail: "We were in a hurry, I'll just say that."

At first I'm surprised when Brent reiterates what Courtney said earlier—that neither of them knew what was wrong with him when he returned from Iraq. I thought PTSD was a widely accepted—and totally predictable—condition afflicting almost anyone who experiences combat. Though I have to remind myself that this was 2004 and the public has come a long way in its understanding of mental health disorders since the Bush years.

"I wasn't diagnosed with PTSD for a couple years. I just thought I was weak," he says as we enter a section of trail lined with ponderosa pine trees. "No one goes to mental health [services] when you're in the military, because you could lose your job. And working in prison there's a cop mentality that says, 'Suck it up.' You're a band of brothers and you don't want to be the weak one. Even when you get out, you don't go to mental health [services], because they'll take your gun away, and there's such a stigma—people will look down on you for it."

When he returned, Brent got his master's in environmental science, inspired by the writings of Rachel Carson and Henry David Thoreau. While he didn't understand his panic attacks, nightmares, and fear of his back being exposed, Brent knew he felt better when walking the Rocky Mountain trails. It may be the kind of thing that would inspire eye rolls in those with a "suck it up" mentality in conservative America, but "forest bathing"—which is basically just being in nature, often walking on trails—is increasingly legitimized by science and mental health professionals as an effective treatment for stress and depression.

Though as a newlywed college student with no money and a load of schoolwork, Brent couldn't just live in the mountains full-time, could he?

"When I got back, I was offered a job as a guard in the El Paso County prison," he says. "I went through the whole process, and was about to do it, but then I had to ask myself, 'How can you be a prison guard if you can't handle the smallest confrontation?' I had a constant terror that I was about to be shot, which is not what you want in a prison guard."

Brent instead got work as a park ranger, but found that even citing teenagers for littering was enough to send him into hyperventilation (which he'd then severely criticize himself for). At the same time, he found himself needing a surge of adrenaline just to feel normal, something dangerous that he could still remain in control of. He'd taken to riding his motorcycle at top speeds late at night on winding roads.

"When he was diagnosed with PTSD at the VA, it made a lot of sense," Courtney recalls. He did see a doctor and attended group therapy, but, as Courtney adds, "He's not much of a talker, and so the group therapy didn't work very well for him."

What did seem to do the trick was the psychological cocktail of running, in nature, under the influence of cannabis.

Brent hadn't smoked pot since his days as a metalhead teenager, but once he was free of military drug tests, he was reintroduced to it by a friend, and he found that it was a game changer for his PTSD symptoms.

Around this same time he was also reintroduced to running.

Brent had despised running throughout his high school and military years, but the idea of an ultramarathon appealed to the endless craving for adrenaline pulsing within him. He was pleasantly surprised to discover that running a mountain trail with a headful of THC was a hell of a lot different from gym class or the Air Force PT test.

"I experienced a sense of calmness, a sense of order," he recalls. "Once you get into shape, running becomes very meditative. The rhythm of my feet was very comforting. It put me in a place where I could face the memories without feeling overwhelmed. Without constantly asking myself what I could've done differently. Without trying to deny there's a problem. Without feeling weak."

Slowly, Brent began to notice that he was feeling better not just during the runs but for long periods afterward. Running high was not only his happy place—it also became the altar where he laid his burden down.

"It felt so good to be mentally and physically drained," Brent says, explaining that the need to run 50 to 100 miles illustrates how much emotional pain he was living with. "I needed to exhaust the anxiety. There were days when I'd run in the morning, but it would come back by the afternoon, and I'd have to go out running again."

Essentially, what Brent is describing is a process we all go through. Only for those without PTSD, it's an involuntary, unconscious process—certainly nothing you need to run an ultramarathon for. Trauma isn't only a terrifying experience; it's an overwhelming of our brain's memory-processing systems, preventing someone from being able to put an experience in its proper place (i.e., the past), and so it chaotically pinballs around, often landing in the present (*danger, now, right now, run, danger!*) whenever a similar sensory experience draws it back to the surface (e.g., fireworks = gunfire).

A fascinating study out of Leiden University in the Netherlands suggests that anandamide is an essential component of our memory processing systems—explaining why endurance running aids PTSD recovery. When thoughts of traumatic experiences are accompanied by a flood of negative emotion, anandamide can calm these systems, allowing the higher functions of our conscious brain to steadily process the memories.

Another study shows that when aerobic exercise is prescribed for patients battling severe depression, it's anandamide that kick-starts the other failing neurotransmitters, like serotonin and dopamine.

In my conversation with the neuroscientist Greg Gerdeman, he mentioned that both cannabis and exercise lead to the growth of new brain cells and new connections between disparate brain regions, also known as neuroplasticity. This, essentially, is the goal of mindfulness therapy, which is the strengthening of the conscious regions of the brain with those governing memory and emotions, allowing us to have a conversation with ourselves and heal the chaos of mood disorders.

When I ask Courtney about the biggest change she's seen in Brent since he began running high, she says that "he asks for what he needs now." This implies that Brent is more vocal about his emotions and that for the first time his neurally integrated brain has the ability to deduce what's going on and to ask himself what he needs to fix it.

Cannabis has become a popular treatment for veterans suffering from PTSD around the globe, with studies showing it has led to a reduction in alcohol and opioid abuse in veterans. When I reported on the first sale of recreational pot in the world, in January 2014, it was Iraq war vet Sean Azzariti who was chosen to make the first purchase, a necessary wet blanket on the otherwise celebratory occasion, highlighting the VA's prohibition against doctors recommending cannabis for combat veterans.

Throughout the nation, thousands of PTSD-stricken veterans have found relief in cannabis, yet are prosecuted alongside rapists and murderers for possession of their medication. As I'm running high with Brent on this Colorado trail, PTSD-suffering Iraq veteran Sean Worsley is being sentenced to five years in one of America's most violent prisons, in Alabama, for possession of marijuana that was legally prescribed to him in Arizona.

These are the details swimming behind my eyes as I jog along this trail, my attention dancing around how Brent Connell fits into my book, whether I've chosen the right training plan for my next race, whether I should buy an earthship. And then my left knee buckles after being slammed by a pair of goat horns.

I look behind me and two pairs of cute yet mischievous eyes are staring me down.

"They can be very rude," Brent says, shooing them away from me. The two goats scatter but keep their eyes on me. "They're testing you. They want to see if they can dominate you."

We jog some more, and my attention drifts to my upcoming travel plans, my finances, and when the next season of *Ozark* will drop. Then another set of goat horns rams into my thigh.

It feels hard enough to leave a bruise, giving me a visceral understanding of how heavy and powerful these young goats are. I'm starting to realize I'm not getting out of this without a challenge.

We're still running uphill, and while the goats are panting, they're remaining a few paces ahead, looking back at me from each side of the trail. *All right,* my stoned mind telepathically says to these goats, *you wanna see what I got? Are you sure?*

Bring it, I see their eyes say.

I've been training pretty hard and am curious myself what I can do. I pull in a few giant breaths, dig my toes into the soft earth, and propel myself up this rocky incline. I sprint past the goats, but they catch up quickly, shooting their horns inches from my knees. I leap from rock to rock, over fallen trees, splash through puddles, but the goats stay on me. I find another gear of energy and take a big lead just before we reach the top.

I immediately spin around, stomp my foot, and shout, "Ha!"

The goats stop and back up, panting and digging at the ground.

Then they slowly go around me as I taunt them like the petulant child I am.

When I turn around, I am struck by the gorgeous site of snow-capped mountains and immediately wonder how much distance and elevation we just ran, and at what pace. It's then that I realize I didn't even wear my Garmin watch on this run. I was so captivated by this circus of animals and trails that I never thought to calculate this run into my training plan.

And goddamn, wasn't that fun? I tell myself.

I honestly can't remember the last time I enjoyed a run so much. For the last few months I've been so obsessed with the numbers, I've essentially neutered the playfulness of running with the dull blade of math, leaving the experience as wild and adventurous as cleaning my bathtub. How could I have let this happen?

I suddenly understand why Brent hated running so much in the Air Force and the appeal of running alongside animals. There's no way these goats would let me get away with listening to podcasts or even music while running alongside them. They wouldn't allow my attention to drift toward my book or some boring training plan. It makes sense for someone in danger of getting lost in thought, particularly terrifying thoughts, to want some goats on hand. They ground you in the playful present.

Brent never listens to music or anything when he runs.

He tells me about the meditative practice of ChiRunning, which, like it sounds, is basically paying very close attention to various aspects of your body and the world around you while running. This is diametrically opposed to how most Americans (and myself as of late, I'm ashamed to say) experience their exercise routines. We hypnotize ourselves with screens and earbuds, or mentally undress others at the gym, in order to segregate our minds from the experience. This often leads to burnout, as you haven't given your mind the opportunity to properly take in the experience with all its faculties.

Just as PTSD robs the brain of its ability to process an experience, we voluntarily engage similar mechanisms when divorcing our brains from our bodies during exercise. We don't all have access to a pair of rambunctious goats, but cannabis (or canines) can also be an effective aid for staying in the present. Brent, like countless other cannabis athletes I've spoken with, talks of getting "dialed in" to his running while under the influence. It doesn't take you away from the experience—just the opposite. It makes you pay ultra close attention to it, utilizing playfulness and curiosity (as opposed to arduous determination) to get the most out of it.

The same principles of ChiRunning apply to high running and goat running: *Lean into the experience.* And if you don't, you just might get a horn up your tuchus.

Later that night Brent and I eat some psychedelic mushrooms he's grown himself.

We sit by a crackling fireplace in his living room, discussing everything from evangelical support for Trump to whether the human immune system has a consciousness independent of our own. The next morning we eat scrambled eggs laid by his chickens, and as I drive off toward my next interview, I find myself deeply envious of Brent Connell's life. Or at least the second half of it.

CHARIOT OF FIRE

André Kajlich has no memory of losing his legs.

On December 6, 2003, he was a hard-partying American student studying chemistry abroad at Charles University in Prague. One night, a half gallon of vodka was being passed around at a party, and André—always wanting to take things to the next level—accepted the bottle, drained it, and blacked out. Weeks later he woke up in an ICU with a punctured lung, injured liver, several broken ribs, and dozens of tubes coming out of him. And though they still felt like they were there, he was missing his left leg at the hip and his right leg at the upper thigh.

It was later explained to him that the morning after the party, he passed out on the tracks of a busy subway station and was crushed by an oncoming train. After a two-month struggle, he was lucky to be alive but was also having trouble with how to define that word now that he'd lost his legs.

"What am I gonna do now?" he told his mother in a morphine haze while being airlifted to his hometown of Seattle, where more surgeries awaited him. "What can I do with my life after this?"

Seventeen years later, I'm straining to keep up with André, leaping over rocks and tree branches, trying to stay close enough to get his words on my recorder as we ascend this trail.

Following my stay with Brent and his goats at the earthship, I hopped in my rental van and drove 1,300 miles to Santa Rosa, California, eager to meet one of the most hard-core wheelchair athletes in the world. My body is stiff after twelve hours in the car, but I think even if I were in perfect condition, I'd still feel challenged to ascend this steep, technical trail.

With his thickly muscled upper body, square and stubbled jaw, and trucker's cap, André looks like he could be a burly MMA fighter—at least from the waist up. He's riding in a three-wheeled chair he designed and welded himself, which keeps him low to the ground and stabilizes him on rocky terrain, while he powers those wheel rims with his massive upper-body strength.

Despite knowing how disabled people feel about being pitied or treated as helpless, I have to admit I'm very nervous that André is about to get hurt. Every few minutes his chair tips dramatically to one side or gets pinched between two large rocks, and I impulsively think, "Help him!"

But every time he tips over, André gracefully pushes off the ground with one thickly calloused hand and rights himself. When his chair gets stuck, he simply grabs the sides, hops, yanks it free, and keeps rolling. We encounter joggers and cyclists who can't believe their eyes, seeing a man in a wheelchair several miles up a technical trail. They cheer him on and, while André waves, nods, or says thanks, he rolls his eyes once they're gone.

"I know they mean well," he says, "but I have a hard time not feeling condescended to, considering this trail isn't much of an accomplishment for me."

I could spend the rest of this book listing André's accomplishments, but for now I'll just stick with the highlights. After dominating wheelchair athletic events like the Panamerican Paratriathlon and becoming the USA Triathalon Paratriathlete of the Year, he moved on to more challenging races, winning the National Ironman 70.3, twice landing silver at the International Triathlon Union World Championships, and setting the record at the SoCal Cycling Challenge 400.

During the triathlons—which traditionally involve swimming, biking, and running—André uses his wheelchair for the running section, a chair with a hand crank for cycling, and only his upper body during the swimming.

The SoCal 400 was a qualifier for the Race Across America,

colloquially known as the world's toughest bicycle race (it's 30 percent longer than Tour de France and must be completed in half the time). Stretching from San Diego to Annapolis, Maryland, cyclists have twelve days to cover 3,100 miles—something never attempted by a hand cyclist. "I slept about ninety minutes a night in the van, then got back on the road for another twenty-four hours, even if it was pouring rain," he says, sounding weary just recalling it. "I had to cover two hundred and sixty-five miles a day to make it. I often hallucinated, or blacked out and woke up in another state. I was at the mercy of my crew."

Ultra road races were certainly challenging, but André was feeling a pull toward nature and was eager to get into some trail races. Trouble was, there was no precedent for wheelchair athletes to race on trails—and therefore no insurance lawyers could sign off on it. Like myself, most race directors assumed that technical trails were too inhospitable for a wheelchair to safely navigate.

Eventually, André convinced the race director of the Brazil 135 that he could handle the race just fine, which was exactly what he did. Once he had an ultra on his résumé, André began slaying the Ironman and Ultraman triathlons, constantly searching for new challenges to feed his restless spirit—which was fueled by cannabis.

"For me, cannabis makes going really hard seem fun and easy. It makes it less painful, both physically and mentally. On the long races that can last days or weeks, you can get bored. But with cannabis, your thoughts become entertainment. Not because they're wacky, but because they're fascinating and stimulate curiosity."

For the last few years, André has been the brand ambassador for Care by Design, a cannabis company specializing in CBD products for athletes, including an alcohol-free THC-infused beer—appealing to athletes because it doesn't cause dehydration. André gave me a bottle of this when we first met in the parking lot—an IPA created in partnership with Lagunitas Brewing. I drank it down, and am now feeling that jolly weightlessness as we enter our fifth mile of the trail.

Between his high-profile racing and working with Care by Design, André has a lot of attention coming his way. These days he can handle navigating the media, the speaking engagements, and the openmouthed stares from hikers as he passes them in a wheelchair. But there was a period of years following his accident when the smallest humiliation would drive him to frozen despair.

"I was really irritable when I came back to the States after my accident," André says. "The morphine they'd had me on in the hospital was brutal to withdraw from, and so I declined the offer to fill up a prescription here. Same with the medication for nerve damage. I didn't want to be on that stuff the rest of my life."

Attempting to navigate both phantom and chronic stabbing pains—each relentless throughout the day and night—without medication was made worse by the existential disorientation of his new life without legs. The crutches, prosthetics, and wheelchair were still foreign objects to him, and he began to stay indoors to avoid the hassle of navigating a world made for the able-bodied. For the first year, André couldn't shake the conviction that he was disfigured, and, like the Elephant Man, feared that his disfigurement would rouse disgust, pity, or bullying from strangers.

"I'd go to the beach with friends but then stop before going in the water, afraid of people seeing me take my prosthetic legs off and crawling the rest of the way to the water," André says as we stop at a scenic point overlooking Santa Rosa, allowing me to grab some much-needed water and deep breaths.

After purchasing a car with hand-controls, André wanted to treat himself to a nice car stereo and began building some speaker cabinets. He drove to Home Depot for materials, but then found himself frozen behind the wheel in the parking lot. It was a busy Sunday afternoon, and André was terrified of all those eyes that would be locked on him when he pulled out his wheelchair, lowered himself into it from the truck, and then wheeled inside the most alpha-male retail store in America, feeling like half a man.

"This is ridiculous," he told his reflection in the rearview mirror. "You can't live like this."

Looking for new ways to engage with the world, André reconnected with some high school friends who still lived down the street. While their ritual of getting stoned and playing video games looked to the world like lazy indulgence, André knew these guys were brilliant and accomplished—one was a physics major who aced his classes, and the other owned a successful insurance agency—and began visiting their house a few times a week to get high and enjoy the company of old friends.

"I didn't know why at the time, but I always felt better when leaving there. Getting high relieved my physical pain and helped with the nerve damage, but the biggest thing was I just felt better about life. Things felt easier."

When he confessed this "drug use" to his therapist (remember, this was 2005 and weed was still very much illegal in Seattle), he was surprised to hear her say, "It sounds like this is really helping you. I think you should keep using it."

When I ask how it helped him, André stops his chair and thinks for a minute.

"There was this night when we all went out to a movie—I think it was *March of the Penguins*. We were late, and the theater had this weird entrance right up front, next to the screen. The place was packed, and everyone was facing us as we looked around, trying to find a seat."

André was using forearm crutches at the time, and typically would've been horrified at all those faces watching him clumsily ascend the aisle, squinting in the darkness to find a seat. But this time, André had consumed some cannabis with his friends beforehand, and suddenly this typically nightmarish scenario became fun, like some kind of game.

"I told myself, 'It's not like they have lasers in their eyes. Nothing happens when they stare.' The cannabis helped make connections in my mind that led to new thinking patterns and made creative strategizing a lot of fun. This would help me a lot when I got into endurance racing and would have to navigate mental barriers."

Soon, cannabis became not only an essential treatment for his pain but a way to change his perception of any given task. Suddenly his wheelchair transformed from a prison to a playground, and he found himself riding it several miles a day to and from work, smoking a joint while listening to Romanian folk music or African blues on his headphones.

"I'd be really tired or unmotivated after a long day at work, then I'd get high and feel rejuvenated. I'd come home and want to work out some more."

Being able to flip the script on life's challenges gave André a hunger to explore where his limits really existed. When he'd first returned home with no legs, the world seemed to be filled with activities that were no longer for him, places he couldn't go without feeling self-conscious. But now it seemed like there was literally nothing he couldn't accomplish, starting with entering a crowded movie theater and continuing on to the most challenging ultra and Ironman races in the world.

"I was still getting an 'isn't this cute' look from other participants at the start of the races, but I didn't care. I wasn't there to compete against anyone but myself."

Once it seemed like he had climbed every mountain, André started looking around for the next challenge that would test his limits. He began to wonder whether these races—with their aid stations, marked trails, and cheering fans—were just a little too cushy. "After a while, an Ironman competition became like an easy training day for me."

In fact, maybe even starting at the base of a mountain was a bit soft.

"I got the idea that it would be cool to try and go from the lowest point on Earth to the very highest, on each continent," he says. Though for André, this was much more than a macho stunt. Suddenly he wasn't just racing for himself anymore.

"I'd learned about disabled kids in places like Ghana, where they were abandoned and stigmatized, because people thought they were cursed. At the same time, there was a lot of optimism around me as a disabled person. I felt so lucky, and I wanted to try and help improve others' situations. And since no one had attempted this feat before—wheelchair or not—I knew there was an opportunity for this to raise some money, change some people's opinions, and take us around the world, putting us in contact with disabled kids, getting them adaptive equipment and some new role models."

After establishing the Lowest to Highest Foundation, André went on the lookout for a couple of disabled athletes to join him on this quest. He met Mohamed Lahna and Lucas Onan at the Million Dollar Challenge, an 800-mile bike ride from San Diego to San Francisco. Both were very accomplished paratriathletes and were excited to meet someone as crazy as they were.

"The three of us got to talking afterward and realized we were kindred spirits in our outdoor adventures, pushing ourselves beyond our perceived limits," Lucas—who was born with an underdeveloped left arm—would later tell me. "André had achieved so much that no one thought was possible. It was really inspiring for kids to see. I think of him like some kind of Viking."

"André doesn't need to prove himself to anyone," adds Mohamed, who is missing his right leg. "He loves to inspire kids and their parents, as we do, but the challenges are about proving something to ourselves, and there's healing in that."

André had an easy time selling Lucas and Mohamed on his fucked-up idea of traversing each continent from the lowest to the highest points, as it spoke to their craving for unexplored challenges. A short time earlier, Mohamed ran the Marathon des Sables, possibly the toughest footrace on Earth, at 156 miles through the Sahara. But even that race, as dangerous as it was, had some structure to it.

This time, the three disabled athletes would be on their own.

"Our first attempt would be in South America, going from three hundred and forty-one feet below sea level to nearly twenty-three thousand feet," André tells me as we sit in his backyard, getting stoned. "The three of us biked sixteen hundred miles through the desert in the first four days, sometimes riding until two a.m., until we reached the base of the mountain. Then we started to climb."

It was at moments like this that Andre's perspective shift—via cannabis—served him well in turning a grueling challenge into a game of playful strategizing.

Over a period of weeks the three of them learned how to complement one another, realizing that where one was weak, the other was strong. Having only one functioning arm, Lucas didn't have a free hand while biking to drink or eat, so Mohamed would feed him and pour water into his mouth as they rode. André was the strongest cyclist, so when the headwind got too much, the other two could draft off him. When the mountain became too much for even André's custom chair, "he would hop down and do his gorilla walk while I'd carry his bike," says Lucas.

"The climb was very challenging," remembers Mohamed. "Lucas was the only experienced climber, but André was so determined.

Seeing his power as he climbed up a mountain . . . I thought I knew everything about disabilities, but this blew me away."

Around eighteen thousand feet of elevation, however, André found his limits.

He'd had to ditch his bike at sixteen thousand feet and utilize his upper-body strength to claw his way up the rest of the mountain. After a certain point, altitude sickness began to take hold. As the experienced climber, Lucas had a physiology accustomed to breathing near the sky, but the other two were in bad shape.

André had a splotchy tongue and couldn't stop throwing up— which was profoundly dangerous, considering the calories he was burning and the dehydration that comes with exercising in thin air. After several failed attempts, the group was forced to turn around just four thousand feet short of their goal.

Like when he did the Race Across America, André did not bring any cannabis with him on this trip. In both cases, there were so many variables to juggle, and adding the transport of an illicit substance was just too much of a hassle (if not a serious crime).

Though looking back, André can't help but wonder if a little cannabis might've been just the ticket when he was suffering on that mountain. There had been plenty of endurance races—or long training sessions—where he'd felt completely spent physically, emotionally, and mentally, and then he'd spark a joint, take a few hits, and suddenly it was a new day, a fully restored André.

Living in Colorado, I've heard arguments both for and against cannabis use when experiencing altitude sickness. The typical symptoms include headaches, vomiting, and loss of appetite—all of which cannabis has been shown to effectively treat. Too much THC, however, could further the disorientation, leading to more vomiting, which is why some caution against this treatment. Though a low-THC, high-CBD product could possibly have settled André's stomach enough to keep water and food down, potentially reviving his system enough to continue those last four thousand feet.

While it was certainly disappointing, none of the three athletes was discouraged by falling short of their goal. In separate conversations, all three of them tell me that, just like with every other race they've done, they're not out to prove anything to anyone but themselves (and maybe the disabled kids they meet along the way). The only competition happens internally, and that's a game where they set their own rules.

For André, cannabis has a role to play in this as well.

"It can help me have a lack of concern about things not going the way I planned, or confronting failure. The value of trying these things isn't in winning—it's being in the moment. And cannabis helps me find that."

At the current moment, these three are planning their next lowest-to-highest adventure, which will be sponsored by Care by Design, the cannabis company André works for. They're aiming to tackle Europe, where the Caspian Sea is the established lowest point, but there's some debate whether Mount Elbrus or Mont Blanc is the highest peak. Just to be sure, André aims to climb both.

While he continues with his pull-ups, push-ups, rowing, cardio, and a whole galaxy of core workouts, strengthening his body to withstand any environmental challenges, the research and development team at Care by Design are using him as their own guinea pig, feeding him a variety of edibles, tinctures, and vaporizers to gauge how it affects his mood, energy, and performance as an athlete.

The cannabis industry still has a long way to go in its effort toward dialing in products for the vast variety of ailments affecting athletes. In the meantime, André is having a blast testing the limits of modern science and his own extraordinary body.

COME OUT AND PLAY

Driving back to my hotel from André's house, I can't stop asking myself how I wound up writing a book about sports.

For years, my identity was wrapped up in actively *hating* any kind of athletic games. I wasn't just indifferent. I went out of my way to tell people how much I loathed the wide world of sports. The whole concept of team spirit confused the hell out of me. *What do you mean, we won the game?* I often wondered when people used this phrase. Beyond the fact that *you* had no part in the game, the idea that any team represents its home city just baffles me. The players are shipped in from all over the country, and the managers, coaches, and owners aren't likely to be locals either. And, similar to religious affiliation, no one *chooses* a team to represent them. It's entirely decided by the geography of your birth. Whenever I've been forced to drink in a sports bar, I often have no idea what team to root for, or even understand how they score points (leading me to jump with fear every time the bar unexpectedly explodes with screams and applause).

Though, if I'm forced to be honest, I understand that prissy rants like these are really just me not dealing with my emotional baggage from growing up as a sensitive artist surrounded by alpha-male, sports-obsessed meatheads who worked their biceps by picking me up by my underwear. It's shortsighted and unfair and I need to get over it.

And I know this because today I love running more than anything.

Which is fucking crazy.

Had this passion for running been inside me all along, or was it simply implanted in me, like the face-hugger from *Alien*, when I swallowed that 10-milligram edible?

When I get to my hotel room, I take a few puffs from a pen vaporizer and listen to the Belle and Sebastian song "The Stars of Track and Field," which has been in my head all day. I was first introduced to this song in 1998, and it blew my mind to hear an effeminate indie-rock band wax poetic about the tender virtues of running. "You only did it so you could wear / Your terry underwear / And feel the city air / Run past your body," frontman Stuart Murdoch sings. Around the same time, I watched my teenage crush Jared Leto star in the Olympic biopic *Prefontaine*, and again found myself feeling some whimsical pull toward running. The desire was always there, trapped beneath cultural assumptions about the type of people who ran (i.e., jerks), and it took cannabis to help me set all that aside for a moment and recognize how much fucking fun it was.

Putting my feet up on the hotel room desk, I lean back and think about how common my story is.

If he'd never gotten high, Roger Boyd may never have thought to spend weeks riding his bike around the English countryside (and eventually the world). Before cannabis, Jerry Dunn and Brent Connell associated running only with shouting drill instructors (a culture that uses exercise as a form of punishment, never something you embrace for your own pleasure). Until he began getting high with his friends, André Kajlich associated his wheelchair only with humiliation and limitation.

What did these endurance activities become after cannabis? Playful.

It's a word commonly associated with childhood, and this underscores a dangerous trend in modern life for adults. Our obsession with utility, ambition, and productivity above all else is, ironically, wildly counterproductive, as modern science shows us that we're far more useful in a state of play.

"Nothing lights up the brain quite like play," says Dr. Stuart

Brown, founder of the National Institute for Play, whose TED talk I look up on my computer while getting stoned in this hotel room. "Three-dimensional play fires up the cerebellum and puts a lot of impulses into the frontal lobe, the executive portion of the brain. It aids in contextual memory, and on, and on, and on."

This makes me think of that scene in *The Sandlot* where the new kid on the baseball field can't seem to catch or throw to save his life. "You think too much," Benny "the Jet" Rodriguez admonishes him. "You gotta stop thinking and have fun. If you were having fun, you would've caught that ball."

The message here isn't a plea for self-care, or the need to relax so that you don't make others uncomfortable. He's saying you're *better at the task* if you're playful. This is often what trips people up with major life obstacles like finances, sex, or working with a team: When it's scary and seemingly impossible, it's harder. When you're creative and having fun, it's easier. (Though getting to the fun part isn't always so easy.)

Like children, animals constantly engage in play throughout their lives, no matter their age. This would explain why Brent Connell enjoyed running with goats so much, and why I suddenly decided to give it a try after watching Iggy have the time of his life sprinting in the park.

I and so many others I've spoken with achieved some type of healing through cannabis-fueled playfulness, but that was never the objective. We were just doing it because—after ingesting cannabis— it became fun to move our bodies. All the mental and physical benefits were just serendipitous side effects, in the same way that a pleasant night's sleep happens to heal your brain and body. But most of us fall asleep each night just because it feels good to sleep. To think of running as a necessary form of health care would potentially ruin its playful undercurrent.

"If its purpose is more important than the act itself, it's probably not play," says Dr. Brown. "Play is born out of curiosity and exploration."

But why does cannabis facilitate this?

Wrestling with my own thumping (THC-fueled) curiosity, I pull out my phone and make another call to Dr. Ethan Russo, the neurologist and cannabis science expert I mentioned in the last chapter. (There aren't many advantages to being a freelance journalist, but being able to ring up experts whenever you get a curious itch about something certainly is one of them.)

"There hasn't yet been research looking into what regions of the brain are stimulated in relation to play when consuming cannabis," he tells me. "But what we do know is that cannabis clearly changes people's perspective on things. [Famed cannabis scientist] Dr. Lester Grinspoon said that when he was facing a thorny problem, he would think about it sober, then think about it high, and that was a way to gain two different perspectives on things."

Oasis songwriter Noel Gallagher has had a similar tradition when listening to playbacks of songs he's recorded, finding that he also has a different perspective on the music when high.

Ethan tells me that he's never experienced a natural runner's high. "But," he says, "when consuming cannabis in the past I've found a strong desire to go out and walk, particularly in nature. My research has found that [cannabis-induced playfulness] often occurs in activities that require a certain rhythm. I've heard from countless skiers who talk about having a bad day on the slopes, and then they consume cannabis and they ski much better. Quite clearly one of the things people like about cannabis is distancing themselves from emotional and physical pain, the ability to compartmentalize things that allows a difference in perspective on one's situation. So those skiers may have a reduction in anxiety about the advancing slope and are able to be in the moment and enjoy it more."

This reminds me of something that German scientist Johannes Fuss told me, that singing and masturbation—two of the most playful activities a human can engage in—both lead to increases in anandamide. Anecdotally, there is strong evidence that cannabis can turn an otherwise painful or mundane chore into a playful challenge. (I can't tell you how many people I've met who love to get stoned before cleaning their house—myself included.) The physical strain and exhaustion are still there, but the way the brain processes that stimuli has shifted.

"What cannabis has over other painkilling medications is that it impacts both the physical and emotional aspects of pain," Ethan says. "People with chronic pain report that when they use cannabis, they can still feel the pain, but they react to it differently. And nothing else does that."

Obviously, a reduction in pain is integral to the playful experience, and probably goes a long way toward explaining why we associate this state with children, who typically don't suffer from the same pains as adults when moving their bodies. When I get up the next morning and drive from Santa Rosa to Las Vegas, I'll be meeting someone who will teach me just how detrimental pain can be to the playful spirit.

And how much conservative America views cannabis-induced playfulness as a threat to its way of life.

GANJA GYM

In the winter of 2012, Jennessa Lea was waiting to die.

She sat slumped in a wheelchair, drifting between pain and numbness as conflicting armies of pharmaceuticals warred within her system. Nearly every nerve in her body would get its chance to scream throughout the day, as a rare disorder weakened her joints to the point where they randomly dislocated with the slightest movement. This was not helped by her accelerating obesity, but at the time fast food was one of the few pleasures Jennessa experienced in a day.

A Minnesota blizzard raged outside as she watched her five-year-old daughter, Isobel, playing at the foot of her wheelchair. Buzzing guilt radiated throughout Jennessa, as a single tear rolled down her cheek.

Isobel deserved better, she told herself. Isobel deserved to have a mother she could be proud of. But Jennessa felt so helpless. The pain, and the drugs used to treat the pain, left her a mindless jellyfish in that wheelchair. She was able to pull it together enough to give Isobel the basics of food, clothes, school, and home. But after that, she was too wiped out for even the smallest conversation.

She wished Isobel's father were around to take care of her.

Or anyone who could provide her a stable, loving home for the next thirteen years. That way, Jennessa would be free to check out from this body that had tortured her for as long as she could remember. She dreamed of the freedom to commit suicide like others dream of winning the lottery.

While she'd had hypermobility—and pain—in her joints her whole life, the problem worsened so badly after she gave birth that Jennessa could hardly move without a shocking level of agony. At the same time, all the tendons, muscles, and cartilage holding her joints together only weakened with inactivity. So the problem was getting worse the less she moved, but the pain was manageable only if she didn't.

Jennessa wouldn't be formally diagnosed with Ehlers-Danlos syndrome, a disease that attacks the body's collagen proteins, which make up the connective tissue throughout the body, until 2013.

Before that, doctors were throwing every medication in their arsenal at the problem, which eventually grew to include oxycodone, morphine, Xanax, Valium, Ambien, Seroquel, Adderall, and Zoloft.

The disease impacted more than just her joints. All the connective tissue throughout her organs, skin, blood, and bones was weakened, resulting in a whole galaxy of pain and complications. She gritted her teeth through physical therapy, the pain nearly driving her to madness and leaving her wiped out for the rest of the week.

As she sat in her chair watching her daughter play, a news story came on the TV about Rick Simpson Oil, a cannabis concentrate that its creator and namesake claimed had cured him of skin cancer. Jennessa had been hearing a lot of stories about all the various ailments cannabis successfully treated, and she figured she had nothing to lose.

Though it turned out, she did.

After she obtained Rick Simpson Oil on the black market (Minnesota had no medical marijuana program at the time), the discovery of cannabis in her system put up a red flag on her medical chart, and suddenly Jennessa was cut off from all her medications. Jennessa didn't think her pain could be any worse, but withdrawing from some of the most potent opioids and benzodiazepines on the market was a transcendent level of hell no one should be forced to endure.

And yet . . . the cannabis oil was really taking effect.

Once she recovered from the constant vomiting, lethargy, insomnia, muscle aches, and anxiety from the pharmaceutical withdrawal, Jennessa felt her pain symptoms begin to dissipate. She was far from cured, but the brief respite from pain gave her some hope that there was a way forward. It was scary to have hope, but the maternal instinct to be a good role model and provider for Isobel allowed her to push through the fear.

Her joints couldn't handle any form of impact exercise, but she found she was able to perform light workouts in a pool. Even this would've been too painful before the cannabis oil, but now she was able to strengthen the muscles around her joints enough to slowly advance out of the pool into low-impact workouts, and, following a knee surgery, then run a 5K every day. She ditched the processed foods, began eating nutritiously, and saw her depression and anxiety dissolve. For years Jennessa had suffered heart palpitations due to a valve that never closed properly (caused by a lack of collagen). An echocardiogram now revealed the valve was strong and closing just fine.

Two years later Jennessa was down one hundred pounds, off all prescription drugs, and could take Isobel hiking or kayaking on the weekends.

"Being in nature was very healing for both of us," Jennessa tells me years later, as the two of us stroll through Red Rock Canyon outside Las Vegas. "Not just for our bodies, but our minds and souls. Our quality of life is vastly different."

It's profoundly hot, but Jennessa is comfortably navigating these trails in yoga pants, a tank top, and a CamelBak. Her tattooed arms appear strong and graceful, showing no sign of injury. Her bright-green eyes sparkle above rosy cheeks and a pierced nose, framed by purple highlights in her long, flowing hair. She speaks with energy and passion as we hike through this canyon, and I'm having a difficult time picturing her one hundred pounds heavier, wheelchair-bound, and dying—both physically and spiritually.

Jennessa credits CBD with aiding her muscle recovery, which is backed by research showing the cannabinoid reduces not only inflammation but muscle spasticity, allowing the tissue to heal. It's also been shown to be an effective sleep aid, which is the time when muscles repair and grow.

In 2014, Jennessa told her story to the Minnesota state legislature, which was considering a bill to legalize medical marijuana. "This plant gave me a quality of life I never thought I'd achieve," she tells me. "It wouldn't be right to keep that to myself if other people could benefit from it."

The legislation passed, though it was one of the most restrictive medical marijuana programs in the country, allowing for only a limited number of products for a small list of conditions—neither of which met Jennessa's needs.

In 2016 Jennessa and Isobel moved to Denver, where recreational cannabis had been legal for two years. Integrating herself into the cannabis community, Jennessa realized she was far from the only one who liked to get high and work out. Perhaps there was a market for a cannabis gym?

It's an endeavor that had been attempted by 420 Games founder Jim McAlpine as well as triathlete Clifford Drusinsky, though the fuzzy regulations of cannabis events (not to mention the unprecedented liability insurance) made it too risky for any investors to back. The constitutional amendment legalizing cannabis in Colorado made it illegal to consume the substance "in public"; consumption was legal only in "a private residence."

Though in 2016, there wasn't a legal precedent to clearly define what "public" and "private" meant in relation to cannabis consumption.

Cannabis entrepreneur Jane West was hosting marijuana brunches in 2014 when one of her events was raided by Denver special task force agents in tactical gear, who were screaming and pointing automatic rifles at tables of soccer moms eating vegan quiche. After several similar incidents, event organizers realized they could turn preorder tickets into RSVPs, turning their parties into private events where the government couldn't intervene.

Jennessa felt like she'd jumped through all the necessary hoops when she converted her spacious basement into a gym and launched Break the Stigma Fitness. She was operating on private property just outside Denver in the town of Wheat Ridge. Guests would RSVP beforehand and sign liability waivers. She paid all necessary taxes, and even discussed every aspect with the local business center, which said that she'd covered all her bases and issued her a business license.

The demand was instant and overwhelming.

While most gyms offer a sterile, isolating atmosphere, often intimidating for those who don't fit the cultural stereotype of a gym rat, Jennessa designed Break the Stigma more like a nightclub, with chill, colored lights, a wall of mirrors, and a disco ball. For twenty-eight dollars, guests could attend a kickboxing, yoga, or high-intensity interval training (HIIT) class, or do their own thing with the variety of standard gym equipment, followed by educational classes on how to properly medicate—or just supplement a workout—with cannabis.

Bongs, pipes, and dab rigs lined the walls, and all sorts of edibles, concentrates, and flower were available free of charge (an essential legal component to the operation), thanks to a handful of cannabis sponsors.

A majority of the guests were new to the gym experience, or even to exercise in general. Like myself and others in this book, many participants had previously considered exercise a tedious obligation, but the cannabis and the atmosphere facilitated a perspective shift, turning exercise into the most enjoyable part of their day.

After receiving some publicity about her own miraculous transformation, Jennessa was inundated by people who also felt caged in their own pain-filled bodies and were discovering physical release through cannabis fitness—as well as a new community of friends.

"People with chronic pain or disability live at home a majority of their life," Jennessa explains, getting a little choked up, "and providing a space where they can share their stories with each other was huge. A lot of them were new to gyms, or hadn't worked out in a long time, because they never felt like there was a place for them somewhere like Gold's Gym."

For a year Break the Stigma was on track to become a lucrative business with a lot of growth potential. Isobel was proud of her mother's entrepreneurial drive, and Jennessa worked all the harder thinking she might have a secure business to pass on to her daughter when she's grown.

While the press she got from left-leaning outlets like *NowThis* and the *Denver Post*'s pot publication, *The Cannabist*, garnered her a plethora of new clients, when the local Fox station did a profile on Jennessa—featuring her ripping a bong surrounded by grandmothers and college kids under Burning Man–like lights—there was an immediate pushback from the think-of-the-children suburbanites who simply wouldn't stand for it.

The next day Jennessa discovered her business license had been revoked.

The citation was for operating a "cannabis club" and selling cannabis without a license. Jennessa balked at both charges, because she was operating within a private residence and never charged customers for any cannabis products. What infuriated her most of all though, she says, was that the business center that revoked her license is the same one that approved her in the first place, knowing every detail of the operation. (The Wheat Ridge Business Center failed to respond to multiple emails on this matter.)

Jennessa never learned why they changed their mind but assumes it was because some outraged neighbors saw her on the evening news.

"I didn't have the money to hire a lawyer to fight it," she says, anger rising in her voice. There was hope that lawyers in the cannabis industry would come to her aid, but before they could, her landlord— who was also aware of the operation from the beginning—evicted

Break the Stigma Fitness. Jennessa found herself without an income, and therefore didn't have the means to fight for her small business.

Looking back, it does seem tragic that Jennessa was persecuted while so many others thrived under the same business model. I was teaching a cannabis creative-writing class, Lit on Lit, around this time, and we operated under the same RSVP ticketing and free-weed-with-purchase model as Break the Stigma. We were never the target of any outrage or legal persecution.

Though we were in Denver, not the suburb of Wheat Ridge.

With the right legal muscle, funding, and public relations campaign, it's possible Jennessa could've moved her operation to another county and grown her business into something she could've passed on to her daughter. Then again, the fact that no one, to my knowledge, has successfully operated a cannabis gym—at least one known to the public—suggests otherwise.

"I assumed people would see this as a public good," she says as we wrap up our hike and exit the trailhead. "I assumed people were coming around to the fact that cannabis is medicine, it's helping people, and doesn't do the same harm as pharmaceuticals. Break the Stigma was transforming the lives of people who were previously alone and in pain, and I thought that would be seen as something to protect. I guess I was pretty ignorant."

IS CANNABIS A PERFORMANCE-ENHANCING DRUG?

AND IS THAT SUCH A BAD THING?

And God said, Behold, I have given you every herb bearing seed, which is upon the face of all the earth, and every tree. . . . To you it shall be for meat.

—Genesis 1:29

THE SPIRIT OF THE SPORT

I've just arrived home in Denver, and after returning my rental van I immediately hop on a bus for my final session of the University of Colorado Boulder study on cannabis and running. During the bus ride I'm struck by how many signs there are boasting that this or that strip of highway is sponsored by a different cannabis company. Since I don't drive very often, I've never noticed this before, but there are at least a dozen of them.

This makes me wonder: Why are cannabis brands allowed to sponsor roads but not sports games? Why are so many players' careers threatened by a healthy, effective botanical medication that's safer than the opioids pushed on them?

Since the NBA, NFL, MLB, NHL, Olympics, and others are all independent entities, they all have their own policies regarding drug testing and what organizations they get into bed with. The one unifying element between them (at least on this issue) is the World Anti-Doping Agency (WADA), which still lists cannabis as a banned substance for athletes in competition. (Though it did remove non-psychoactive CBD from the list in 2017.)

This designation is the root of the persecution faced by pro athletes caught with marijuana in their systems, like snowboarder Ross Rebagliati, who was stripped of his Olympic gold medal for pot in 1998. Michael Phelps didn't lose any of his twenty-three gold medals when a picture of him ripping a bong surfaced (since he wasn't caught using in competition), but he did lose his sponsorship with Kellogg's, and was suspended for three months by USA Swimming. Even the PGA is not immune to this, recently suspending pro golfer Matt Every for a positive urinalysis, despite his having a medical prescription for the substance.

Why do athletes like Mike Tyson, the Detroit Lions' Calvin Johnson, and the legendary basketball player Cliff Robinson have to wait until they're retired to launch their own line of cannabis products or be endorsed by a cannabis company, like Gary Payton is?

A change in WADA policy would likely curb a lot of this, possibly even allowing teams, athletes, and games to be sponsored by cannabis companies.

When I reached out to WADA to clarify this, I was emailed a form letter explaining that when a substance is banned by the organization, "it must meet two out of three different criteria: 1.) It has the potential to enhance sport performance; 2.) It represents a health risk to the athletes; or 3.) It violates the spirit of the sport." When I replied asking which two of the three cannabis fell under, I was told, "We don't typically declare which of the three conditions have been met when we ban a substance."

Beyond the mystery of where cannabis falls on this, the list itself sends my curiosity snaking in twenty different directions at once. The most urgent question I have is, What the fuck does "the spirit of the sport" mean?

Is opioid use "in the spirit" of football or basketball? Because that definitely qualifies as a health risk, leading to abuse in nearly 30 percent of those who take them. Does numbing an injury with a heroin-like substance so you can perform without pain qualify as a "performance enhancer"?

How is that term even defined?

(Admittedly, before researching this book, my knowledge of how players were abused with opioids was limited to the Paul Walker sports flick *Varsity Blues*.)

In 2011, WADA clarified that cannabis was indeed considered a performance enhancer by its criteria, conducting a study with the (historically anti-pot) National Institute on Drug Abuse (NIDA) that found marijuana "can cause muscle relaxation and reduce/decrease anxiety and tension pain during post-workout recovery . . . and increase focus and risk-taking behaviors, allowing athletes to forget bad falls or previous trauma in sport, and push themselves past those fears in competition."

Those don't necessarily sound like bad things. At least not to me.

If they also violate the "spirit of the sport," does that mean that pain and anxiety are essential components of sports? As we've established, I am not an authority on sports, so I'm not qualified to judge the role of suffering in competition. And I'm out of time to ponder this conundrum, because I now have to go hop into a stranger's van and stick a needle into my arm.

PLEASURE AND PAIN

There's an Orwellian logic to the commonly employed phrase "further study on marijuana is needed before we can legalize it," considering that it's cannabis prohibition itself that is preventing the kind of definitive study needed to push legalization forward.

On the one hand, respected doctors like Andrew Weil proclaim, "We know more about marijuana than we do penicillin. Marijuana has been researched to death, and it is one of the safest drugs known to medicine." And yet, particularly when it comes to cannabis and exercise (and many other questions about the plant), we do not yet have the double-blind placebo trials needed to fully convince the remaining skeptics in the medical science community of its efficacy.

As my bus drives through Boulder, I see a cannabis dispensary every few blocks. As a citizen over the age of twenty-one, I am free to walk in and purchase enough weed to get me high for a month, though if a researcher from the University of Colorado—or any university in a legalized state—wants to conduct a study involving consumption of marijuana, they can't just pick up a few joints at the nearby shop. Since cannabis is still federally illegal, a university would risk losing a great deal of its public funding if it were to bring an illicit substance onto the campus.

It's actually easier to obtain and conduct studies with crack than cannabis.

While Raphael Mechoulam was able to casually ask the police for some confiscated hash when he began conducting his experiments in 1962, today any US scientist wanting some government-sanctioned weed must endure an arduous application process involving the NIH, NIDA, and the Drug Enforcement Administration (DEA).

And while it may not be a formal policy of theirs, history shows us that only studies examining the harms of cannabis—rarely the benefits—receive a green light from these conservative organizations.

When oncologist Donald Abrams wanted to test what he was seeing in his patients—that smoking cannabis relieved the symptoms of "HIV wasting syndrome"—he needed approval from eight different agencies, including the FDA and NIDA, but was initially rejected. "We're the National Institute *on* Drug Abuse, not *for* Drug Abuse," he was told.

After this, he began framing his proposal around how cannabis *worsened* HIV symptoms. This proved successful, and he was able to continue his work in the same manner he'd intended, and he released what was the first of many studies showing that cannabis effectively treated symptoms related to AIDS.*

The DEA has been accused of monopolizing the cannabis science field, since the only institution it allows to legally grow cannabis is the University of Mississippi. What scientists receive from the DEA is either a can of pre-rolled (considerably aged) "marijuana cigarettes" or a brick of freeze-dried flower, requiring a special rehydrator before it can be consumed. While the average recreational flower is around 17 percent THC, the DEA has never allowed the Mississippi scientists to breed anything above 10 percent, or produce any amount of CBD flower. After the plants are harvested and cured, they are ground together—seeds, leaves, everything—resulting in a substance that's quite foreign to the subjects asked to consume it.

CU Boulder neuroscientist Dr. Kent Hutchison—Angela Bryan's husband and partner in the cannabis exercise study I'm participating in—stopped using DEA cannabis years ago when he found it seriously degraded the validity of his research on marijuana users.

"We had them smoke it in the lab, then studied their mood and cognition," he tells me. "And what they told me was, 'That was disgusting. What are you giving me? I would never, ever smoke that stuff.' That's going to bias your research, you're not going to be studying people who are having a pleasant experience, like they do when they go home and smoke their medical-grade marijuana. So the research loses its validity because it doesn't reflect what is happening in the real world."

To circumnavigate this conundrum, Kent and Angela went full-on *Scooby-Doo* and built a mobile laboratory inside a van. It's

....

* You can't overestimate the role cannabis treatment of AIDS in the gay community of San Francisco had on the legalization movement. Many of the products, dispensaries, pioneering legislation, and cultural and scientific shifts around the medical application of cannabis is owed to the courageous efforts of the LGBTQ+ community in the 1980s and '90s.

there to meet me outside a friend's house today in Boulder, where I've just consumed three hits of a strain I was assigned by Kent and Angela's team to pick up myself at a local dispensary (they couldn't legally provide it to me, only arrange the sale). A sample of my blood is taken inside the van, and I'm then quickly driven to the university campus, where I'll run on a treadmill and answer some more questions.

It's a somewhat inelegant dance, mostly orchestrated by lawyers, but it still provides them with scientific data in a semi-controlled environment without risking their federal funding by bringing an illicit product on campus.

The study I'm participating in is concerned with whether cannabis increases our enjoyment of exercise, not necessarily whether it increases performance—so I'm not sure if any of the results would alter WADA's view of cannabis.

As I casually jog in front of a mirror (with a thick strap wrapped around my waist and secured to the treadmill, because someone on the safety board apparently assumed stoned runners are as coordinated as drunken toddlers), I'm wondering whether enjoying exercise is in itself a performance enhancer. And if so, is that antithetical to "the spirit of the sport"?

Is misery an essential cornerstone of sports?

When I was back in California a week earlier, I asked André Kajlich whether cannabis should be considered a performance enhancer. He was quiet for a moment before saying, "You know how some movies are long and slow and take some work to get into, but eventually there's a payoff? Well, that's how endurance sports can be, but cannabis takes the work out of it."

While I understand that André is simply saying that cannabis makes exercise fun from the beginning, I can see how the phrase "takes the work out of it" would irk some alpha males with a no-pain, no-gain sensibility. This makes me wonder if, for some people, overcoming discomfort is "the spirit of the sport."

Though, ultimately, aren't you better at something if you enjoy it?

When I asked Meghan Hicks of *iRunFar* magazine to describe Avery Collins's reputation in the ultrarunning world, she said, "He's known as someone who really enjoys and seeks out the roughest terrains and burliest races, and excels at them." And this isn't because Avery feels no pain. It's because he *enjoys the pain.* "The pain is what you're after," he told me when we first met. "I once threw up blood at an aid station during the HURT100, and when a volunteer asked me if I was okay, I looked up at her, smiled, and said, 'Fuuuuuuck yeah!'"

Neurology shows us that pleasure and pain are not necessarily disparate activities in the brain. Both experiences stimulate a lot of the same brain regions—which goes a long way toward explaining the popularity of BDSM, tattoos, and, really, any endurance sport. Where pain diverts from pleasure is the way it's perceived in the mind, not necessarily the way it's processed in the nervous system. This is why, as Angela Bryan explained earlier, those who are self-motivated to exercise enjoy it, and those who are enduring it because someone insisted they do end up hating it. It's the same activity, just with a different perspective.

And like Ethan Russo said, cannabis can change the way pain is processed in the brain, weakening its emotional punch (or, in Avery Collins's case, increasing it to the point of pleasure).

While running on the treadmill in Boulder, I'm asked about my pain, pleasure, disassociation, and energy every ten minutes. In between those questions, I find myself hypnotized by the full-length mirrors that surround me. I rarely work out at gyms, so the experience of analyzing my gait from all different angles is fascinating to me.

Or at least it's fascinating today.

Just before my road trip I did a run here at the lab without any cannabis in my system, and weirdly enough, I never noticed all these mirrors (and generally found the experience quite boring). Now that I have a headful of cannabis, I'm critiquing my foot placement, my ankle pronation, the angle of my pelvis, the kick of my heels, and my constant battle to lead with my chest and not my head.

Typically, these are the kind of mundane details I don't like to concern myself with during a run, preferring to wrap my attention around swaying trees, running dogs, or a particularly wonderful chord change coming through my headphones. But right now I'm loving the challenge of getting my body into the perfect form. It's taking effort and is difficult, but I'm still fully engaged with my playful, curious side.

Improving my form will keep me from getting injured and allow me to run faster with less effort. Ultimately, I will have *enhanced my performance* without pushing through the mental discomfort of doing something I don't enjoy.

In Malcolm Gladwell's book *David and Goliath*, he describes this phenomenon as "capitalization learning." He uses Tiger Woods as an example of this: someone who was good at something from the start (golf) and got better at it because it's fun to practice things you're already good at. But most high achievers require what he describes as "desirable difficulties," which is pushing through activities that are hard, and mostly remain hard—like reading while dyslexic. In this case, a person will improve at this skill to a greater degree than if they never had the extra challenge, because they had to put forth twice the effort.

Is that, I wonder, *what WADA means by "the spirit of the sport"?*

It would make sense, and be a semi-fair argument against cannabis use in competition (though it would be a terrific argument for why sedentary people should experiment with cannabis and exercise). But as any cannabis-loving endurance athlete will tell you, once you enter into your twelfth, twentieth, or sixtieth hour of a race, there's no level of high you can get that's going to erase the desperate pleas from your nervous system to *please, for god's sake, stop it already!*

Though cannabis can keep your mind in the present moment, allowing you to "forget about the numbers and just run," as Avery Collins says, it's not the only way to achieve this. Ultrarunner Diane Van Deren seemingly came out of nowhere when she became the first female to complete the 430-mile Yukon Arctic Ultra in 2009. She became an ultrarunner only after receiving a frontal lobotomy to stave off seizures, which, unintentionally, stripped her of the ability to perceive time. While racing ultras, she never had any clue whether she'd just started the race or was near the finish line, and this proved to have a profound impact on her level of exhaustion.

This is what endurance athletes mean when they say the sport is 90 percent mental and 10 percent physical. Our pain and level of endurance is often a construct of our brain's cortical regions, which tell us we should stop long before we have to. But does this mean that lobotomies—or meditation, which can also change our relationship to pain and time—should be banned in competition alongside cannabis?

To better understand the world of competition, I hop in a Lyft and head to the Boulder home of triathlete Joanna Zeiger. Before shifting to epidemiology research, Joanna had an epic career in endurance sports, coming in fourth in the 2000 Olympic triathlon, winning the Ironman 70.3 World Championship in record time, and, following her retirement, authoring the book *The Champion Mindset: An Athlete's Guide to Mental Toughness.*

With my punk-rock, anti-competition bias, I expect her message to be some variation of the "tough it up, pussy" rhetoric I endured in high school gym class. But only a few minutes into our conversation I find that we actually have a lot in common—in our approach both to endurance athletics and to cannabis.

"When I was coming up, there was a lot of this go-hard-or-go-home, or go-till-you-blow mentality, but that's not always helpful," she tells me as we sit on her back patio on a sunny Boulder afternoon. "Being kind to yourself, knowing when to stop, and not letting others dictate what you do are essential to mental toughness. A lot of athletes don't have the confidence to go easy—they need big numbers all the time and find their self-worth in the numbers. But athletes need easy days in their training. Small numbers can make a lot of athletes miserable, and when you don't have joy, you don't perform as well."

Like Kent and Angela at CU Boulder, Joanna is looking into the role cannabis can play in shifting the mental perspective (among other things) of athletes with her organization the Canna Research Foundation. "Anecdotally, I've heard from a lot of people who had anxiety about going to the gym, and they'd consume cannabis and it would allow them to put all that aside and do their workout."

Joanna never came in contact with marijuana throughout her career as a professional athlete, which came to an end in 2009 when a volunteer at an aid station didn't let go of the water bottle he handed to her as she peddled away, ripping her from her bike and slamming her to the ground. The fall broke her collarbone and caused permanent structural and nerve damage to her rib cage. It was only in 2018 that she was diagnosed with an auto-inflammatory disease, but the symptoms of that had been plaguing her for more than a decade.

Between these two conditions, Joanna spent years in severe discomfort.

Despite more than nine surgeries and various pharmaceutical

regimens, Joanna was plagued with severe chronic pain, insomnia, nausea, muscle spasms, and difficulty breathing. She was curious about medical cannabis, but the stigma against it in the world of athletics—in addition to her new career as an epidemiological research associate at CU Boulder, where she studied drug abuse in adolescents—left her too embarrassed to apply for a medical marijuana card. Though when it became legal recreationally in 2014, the desperation for a moment's respite from the torture of her body pushed Joanna to overcome her reservations and give pot a shot.

Despite ingesting far too much THC via a transdermal patch (which she would later learn to divvy up into four pieces) and not enjoying the high at all, Joanna had her first pleasant night's sleep in years, and found that it did wonders for her pain, appetite, and muscle spasms. She assumed her doctors would be thrilled to hear about her progress but found that, even in liberal Boulder, "some were so anti-cannabis, they didn't even want to hear about it."

Wanting to know more about why this plant was aiding her in a way no other drug had, Joanna dove into the medical research on cannabis. "I found that there was a huge deficit in the literature. Being an epidemiologist, I was in a position to do some research myself. There was so much anecdotal evidence, but that doesn't translate into doctors believing that it works, or give people the information they need on dosage or disease-specific treatment."

Joanna launched the nonprofit Canna Research Foundation with the intention of assembling data that could be used by medical professionals and patients considering if and how cannabis could be used for various ailments. Its work goes well beyond athletics—it's currently looking into how cannabis impacts allergies, asthma, and inflammatory bowel disease—though as an accomplished athlete and cannabis researcher, she's in a unique position to comment on WADA's prohibition against cannabis.

"Cannabis should be taken off the banned list," she says. "When it comes to steroids or human growth hormones, I don't put cannabis in that category. Is it performance enhancing? Maybe indirectly, because it helps you sleep and eases anxiety and pain. But there are other substances that do the same thing that aren't banned but are more dangerous, like Motrin and other anti-inflammatories. Athletes pop those like candy while they're racing, and that dehydrates you and is harmful to your gut. And there are medications for depression or anxiety that help performance, which aren't banned."

Joanna is very different from most cannabis enthusiasts I meet, who often proclaim marijuana to be the cure to every known ailment with no side effects or potential for addiction. The Canna Research Foundation is just as concerned about the harmful aspects of cannabis as the beneficial ones, and strives for more scientific clarity on where those lines are drawn. But the stigma that keeps cannabis illegal and banned in competition also makes funding and access to volunteer subjects difficult to come by. Joanna says that many scientists and philanthropists are hesitant to publicly wed themselves to this subject, and cannabis consumers are wary of participating even in anonymous surveys about their use.

"For the most part, doctors and the leaders of the cannabis industry don't understand why people are taking cannabis or how it's working for them. Some people seem to need a very high dose, while others only require a small one, some products work for one ailment but not for others, but we don't know why. It's a total quagmire, and people in positions of authority in medicine or sports need to have this information so they can make informed decisions."

After thanking Joanna for her time, I hop on the bus back to Denver, looking forward to a few days of sleeping in my own bed, smoking my own bong, and running in my favorite parks after so many weeks on the road. But on the ride home I look at my phone and discover that in just a few days the Cannabis Science Conference in Portland, Oregon, will feature presentations from a number of pot-loving athletes as well as sports medicine physicians and neurologists.

I am profoundly road weary, but my insatiable curiosity surrounding WADA's prohibition of cannabis in competition and the elusive definitions of the phrases "performance enhancer" and "the spirit of the sport" eclipse my need for domestic comfort, and I find myself booking a plane ticket before the bus even arrives in Denver.

A RETURN TO BALANCE

People have a hard time believing that Janice Knox attended Berkeley in the sixties and was never once exposed to marijuana. But it's true. As a young Black woman pursuing her medical degree in the age of the civil rights movement, there was no room in her life for the flower-power antics of the white kids across the bay.

It would be another thirty-five years—just after she retired from her long career as an anesthesiologist—before Janice was ever (knowingly) in the same room with cannabis. It was 1997, California had recently become the first state to legalize medical marijuana, and Janice was invited to tour a dispensary. She'd expected the clinic to be full of tie-dyed burnouts looking to get high under the ruse of "medicine," but instead she was surprised to find basic-looking grandmothers, lawyers, businessmen, and mothers with very sick children—all suffering from ailments beyond the reach of modern medicine.

Most of them were new to cannabis treatment and had a lot of questions about what type of cannabis was right for their bodies and their conditions, how much to take, and what ingestion method (tincture? edible? smoke?) was best for them. Not only did Janice not know, but she found that the whole medical marijuana operation was woefully unequipped to understand how to guide patients in this process.

Curious, she delved into the research and found a plethora of evidence showing cannabis to be an effective treatment for a profoundly long list of ailments. In fact, there seemed to be a history of medical cannabis use around the world dating back thousands of years—including in this country, until the mid-twentieth century.

So why was it kicked off the American pharmacopoeia?

Looking into the congressional record, she found an epic story of racism, corporate greed, and conservative hysteria that criminalized a popular herbal medication (more on this in the following chapter). Rage boiled in the retired doctor's veins. She thought of the mother she'd lost to breast cancer, and her first son, who'd died of brain damage, and wondered whether cannabis could have effectively treated them.

As she continued to crawl down this medical-marijuana rabbit hole, she began to understand that cannabis wasn't so much a miracle drug but simply the most effective substance for tapping into the endocannabinoid system—which was also mysteriously absent from American medical practice.

Despite the NIH declaring that "the endocannabinoid system is involved in essentially all human diseases," Western medicine apparently didn't value this biological machine in the health-care system. As late as 2013, a survey showed that the endocannabinoid system was taught in only 13 percent of US medical schools (though this has changed in recent years).

"The endocannabinoid system is simply a master regulator. There isn't a single system in the body that it doesn't control, influence, or modulate in some manner," Dr. Janice Knox says, speaking on a panel at the 2019 Cannabis Science Conference in Portland. "Medicine today overspecializes, and so patients are trained to think of their body in different sections—a neurologist for the brain, a cardiologist for the heart—instead of thinking of the body as a whole integrated system. We should be focusing on repairing the endocannabinoid system, not the diseases caused by its imbalance. And cannabis has been shown to be the most effective treatment for that."

Joining Janice on this panel are her two daughters, Jessica and Rachel, and her husband, David Knox, all of who had storied careers in medicine before collectively pursuing the emergent field of endocannabinology—which is basically a realm of medical research and health care that treats the body's endocannabinoid system.

After the panel is over, I approach Janice and ask her why cannabis made me (and so many others) suddenly love running after hating it for so long. Thinking for a moment, she theorizes that this could be due to a hitch in our endocannabinoid system.

"There are a number of things in our modern lifestyle that can throw the endocannabinoid system off balance, like bad food, stress, insomnia, and environmental toxins in our clothes and furniture. And that can lead to deficiencies in endocannabinoids like anandamide, which causes the runner's high," she explains to me, standing in the hallway outside a conference room. "But you can trigger the release of anandamide by ingesting a phytocannabinoid like THC, which would induce the runner's high quicker and more effectively."

This goes a long way toward explaining why something that is integral to our evolutionary reward system, like exercise, has somehow lost its ability to make us feel good. Those with healthy sleep, diet, and exercise habits have equipped their endocannabinoid system with the tools it needs to deliver the natural high from exercise—the production and release of anandamide. When those stuck in the modern lifestyle of deskwork, poor sleep, processed foods, and two hours of high-stress traffic follow that up with a light jog around the park, it's pure agony because their brains aren't capable of producing anandamide.

(Additionally, there are the many psychological barriers that keep people from seeing themselves as worthy of exercise or a healthy body, which often boils down to an anthropological, us-versus-them mentality that reflexively dismisses wellness culture in favor of hedonistic self-destruction as a coping mechanism for one's inferiority complexes. Or at least this was my experience.)

Even more than this, Janice explains to me that anandamide also regulates the release of dopamine, serotonin, and glutamate—all of which make up the evolutionary reward systems that regulate our mood. So just as depression can lead to a spiral of sedentary behavior and consuming shitty food (which leads to more depression), the combination of THC and exercise leads to a deluge of happy chemicals that make you want to run more, which makes you even happier, which makes you want to run more.

But does this make cannabis a performance-enhancing drug?

While Janice Knox is a wizard of the endocannabinoid system, doping regulations in sports is not her expertise.

Luckily, though, the buffet of scientists at this conference offers me a seasoned expert on sports medicine who can shed some light on my athletic ignorance.

"I hear a lot of people say we need to get ready, that cannabis is coming to the world of sports," says sports medicine professor Dr. Jeff Konin, delivering his presentation, titled "Cannabis and Athletics: The Impact in 2020." "Whenever I hear that, I say, 'It's not coming—it's already here.' Athletes are already using cannabis, but there is a stigma that's preventing athletes from being open with their doctors about their use and keeping sports physicians from being educated on what the science is showing us."

After spending thirty years as a physical therapist, Hall of Fame athletic trainer, and sports medicine educator—working at the 1996 Olympics in Atlanta, the University of Rhode Island as chairman of the physical therapy department, and James Madison University as director of sports medicine—in 2018 Jeff Konin encountered the same educational conundrum that Janice Knox experienced in the nineties: a whole lot of people asking about whether (and how) to use cannabis and not knowing how to respond.

In the past he could just advise athletes to not take it, due to its illegality. But once legalization began to sweep the nation and dispensaries started popping up like Starbucks, he found that athletes were using cannabis in training and recovery to great effect—and knew that simply telling them no wasn't an option.

Around this same time, then–Senate majority leader Mitch McConnell signed the Hemp Farm Bill, which federally legalized the mass production of nonpsychoactive CBD products. Suddenly CBD salves and pills were being sold over the counter at Walgreens, offered in coffee shops to supplement drinks, and promoted to every soccer mom and retiree as a healthy alternative to aspirin. Nursing homes boasting CBD treatments were becoming the new fad, but few institutions knew how to regulate it, leading to one grandmother being handcuffed and arrested at Disney World when she was found with a CBD topical oil in her purse.

Jeff Konin was lecturing on concussion treatment for athletes at the time and was fascinated by emerging research showing cannabis could act as an effective treatment for brain damage as well as a neuroprotectant against future damage.* And he was encountering such a deluge of anecdotal stories from athletes about their cannabis-derived relief from pain, anxiety, insomnia, and so many other

....

* In an ironic twist of fate, studies also show that cannabis can act as a neuroprotectant against alcohol-induced brain damage.

ailments that—even though he knew the subject still needed double-blind studies—there was no way all these people could be experiencing the same placebo effect.

"Should I encourage my patients to try some low-dose THC?" he asks during his presentation. "Logically, I thought yes, but legally I couldn't. And that's what made me want to dig into the science. And eventually I started asking, If there's a reasonable treatment or intervention for athletes in need, and it's less harmful than what we're currently giving them, why are we ignoring this?"

With his shaved head and sharp suit, Jeff fits in with the big-business, no-nonsense world of professional sports. The only difference being the tiny gold pin on the lapel of his suit jacket brandishing a subtle yet unmistakable pot leaf. (His license plate also reads PHD420.) When I sit down with him in a coffee shop just outside the convention center, I'm primarily curious if he's as baffled by marijuana's ban in sports as I am.

"If you go to the websites for the NCAA [National Collegiate Athletic Association], WADA, and USADA [US Anti-Doping Agency], they all contradict what one another says in their policies," he explains. "One will say it's banned because it's a performance enhancer. Another says it's not a performance enhancer, there's no evidence it is, but it has adverse side effects, so it's banned. And that's where we are. We don't have everyone on the same page."

Like many of the scientists at this convention, Jeff aims to bridge the gaps between what we know about the efficacy of cannabis treatment and the medical world, which seems largely (often willfully) ignorant of that information. After spending a year immersing himself in the science and speaking with patients, caregivers, researchers, and policy makers, Jeff began a career educating sports medicine providers, as well as athletes and team management, on the safest, most effective uses of cannabis that current evidence has revealed.

While there was an overwhelming interest from athletes for his guidance, the old guard of traditional medicine put up quite a fight. In 2019, Konin supported a proposal that the American Physical Therapy Association create an official collection of educational resources on cannabis, which physical therapists could refer to when their patients asked them about treatment. "They argued for an hour back and forth," he recalls. "And keep in mind this is not to *promote* cannabis, only to collect a body of science on it. In the end it passed, but with only a fifty-to-forty-nine vote."

Jeff says that until those double-blind trials are completed, a lot of physicians and health-care providers aren't going to be on board. Meanwhile, plenty of athletes are using it (because it works) but neglecting to tell their physicians (or straight up lying to them because their career is at stake), which harms the efficacy of their medical treatment.

When it comes to the cost-benefit assessment of cannabis treatment, Jeff says there's one major factor that causes the advocates and the detractors to talk past each other: dosage. Given the biphasic nature of cannabis—meaning that a small dose will deliver euphoria, energy, and focus, and a large dose will result in the opposite— you can have multiple sets of studies showing conflicting results due to variations in how much cannabis participants consumed. So you could have one side arguing that cannabis harms performance (lethargy, anxiety, disorientation), while another side argues that it improves performance (energy, balance, focus), and they can both be right; they're just looking at two very different scenarios.

"Some people will come up to me after my presentation saying, 'Why didn't you include the study from the NCAA showing adverse effects of cannabis?' And I'm like, 'That's because I'm not advocating for high-dose, round-the-clock use since age twelve, which is what those studies are looking at.' The literature is clear that a high dose will result in anxiety, will raise your heart rate. But no one I know of in athletics is promoting anything but low doses, because that's where the benefits are. Trouble is, 'low dose' isn't a specific measurement, and it's different for different people, and we need to find out why."

I've spoken with many ER physicians and general practitioners who say the same thing: that when a patient confesses to use (which they're doing more often now that it's legal), they'll say they take three or four "hits" a day. But the volume of those hits will be different from a pipe, bong, or joint, not to mention the lung capacity of the user. Early in my stoned running days, I certainly encountered moments of taking far too much of an edible and then lethargy and anxiety ruined my run. This is why legal, regulated cannabis products are such a game changer: it's mandated by law that edibles be divided up into 10-milligram servings and be dosed consistently throughout all products. So when I found that 20 milligrams was too much for me, I could easily dial it back to 10.

Given its variety of (sometimes conflicting) effects, cannabis can be difficult to classify as a stimulant, tranquilizer, sedative, or hallucinogen—unlike most drugs—and therefore it's challenging to evaluate it in the same way. Like Janice Knox, Jeff prefers to examine cannabis treatment not through the plant itself but through its impact on the endocannabinoid system. When viewed this way, Jeff says, it's ridiculous to classify it in the same league as other performance-enhancing substances.

"There's clear evidence that steroids will increase the size of your muscle and the power you can produce beyond your natural limits, and that's what makes it a performance enhancer," he explains. "Whereas the endocannabinoid system returns you to a state of balance after you've been depleted. When you don't have endocannabinoids functioning properly in your body, it's no different than a lack of insulin for diabetics or ice for an injury. When I put ice on an athlete's injured ankle, I'm returning that ankle to balance, not taking it beyond its natural limits. It's addressing a medical condition, not enhancing performance."

Jeff doesn't believe that the world of sports medicine and WADA are going to change their tune until heftier science is on the table (which isn't happening until it's federally legalized, which won't happen until there's heftier science on the table, and so on). But he does believe that we're in the middle of a deluge of athletes using cannabis products with promising results, and the more open they are about this, the more recreational athletes will begin using them, creating an even greater demand for his type of work.

"Whatever the pros do—whether it's Breathe Right nasal strips or Gatorade—it trickles down to the rest of the population," he says. "Soon you're going to have more athletes coming out about their use, and even endorsing products, and then it's all over."

While the world of ultrarunning is seeing more and more athletes like Avery Collins and Flavie Dokken sponsored by cannabis companies, and even traditionally conservative road marathons have begun taking on weed sponsors (cannabis growers Cresco Labs became the first when it sponsored the 2014 Chicago Marathon), when it comes to the more traditional sports, we're still a few years away from cannabis brands being as common a sponsor as beer companies, or as normalized an athletic supplement as Gatorade.

As reported at the beginning of this book, there is no shortage of pro athletes secretly consuming cannabis in both their training and recovery. Though at the moment, it's almost exclusively the retired athletes who are coming out as cannabis consumers and embracing this lucrative new industry.

Iconic football names like Brett Favre and Joe Montana have entered the cannabis biz, as have NBA legends like Isiah Thomas,

Magic Johnson, Al Harrington, Cliff Robinson, and Kevin Durant. Baseball MVP Jimmy Rollins has his own line of pre-rolled joints, as does four-time Stanley Cup winner Darren McCarty. And revolutionary feminist soccer player Megan Rapinoe is now sponsored by a CBD brand promoted to athletes.

Many of the products borrowing these celebrity athletes' names and credibility are designed specifically for athletes, mostly for pain relief but some to enhance the workout experience, like Paul Pierce's CBD vaporizer, and AQUAhydrate, the CBD fitness-water company launched by Sean "Diddy" Combs, Mark Wahlberg, and *The Biggest Loser's* Jillian Michaels.

Just like Michael Jordan's unforgettable "I better eat my Wheaties" catchphrase, the unsubtle message of the companies launched by (or paying endorsements to) celebrity athletes is simple: buy our product and excel like these guys. Setting aside any "think of the children!" handwringing for a moment, I can't help but wonder if this trend is oversimplifying—or even trivializing—the science behind cannabis and athletics.

While physicians like Janice Knox, sports medicine experts like Jeff Konin, and researchers like Angela Bryan and Joanna Zeiger are desperate for the kind of hard-hitting studies exploring the divergent effects of various cannabis strains on athletes, the promising yet limited science we do have has been enough for the cannabis industry to lay claim to the biggest names in sports, with some implied product benefits that are rarely scrutinized or regulated.

Obviously, I believe in the power of cannabis to aid athletes in dozens of ways. I just wish the cannabis industry were under greater pressure (or any at all) from consumers to explain what it is about their plants or extraction processes that make their products an ideal supplement for athletes.

On my way to the "Athletes for Cannabis" panel, I run into

Dr. Ethan Russo, the neurologist and cannabis expert I often call. Luckily, he has a couple minutes to answer a few of my questions about athletic-enhancement products in the cannabis industry.

"There are definitely a wide variety of different cannabis types that have different effects, depending on the selective breeding of the plant," he explains as we wait for the athletics panel to begin. "One of the objections I have to modern cannabis breeding is the prominence of high-THC, high-myrcene chemovars."*

If your head is spinning from that last sentence, don't worry.

Ethan Russo tends to speak in a language that's clearly understood by neuroscientists or botanists but that often sounds like gibberish even to those in the cannabis industry—a world he definitely has some reservations about. Ethan is not a fan of smoking cannabis, thinks THC on its own is "a lousy drug," and feels that the extraction process of most edibles and concentrates destroys many of the medical benefits of the plant. Much like Janice Knox's conviction that medical science needs to look at the body as a whole and not individually, Ethan Russo's belief is that there should be more emphasis on the cannabis plant as a whole and not just isolating THC or CBD on their own—particularly since CBD has been shown to counteract the anxious effects (i.e., "the fear") of excessive THC.

As strange as it may sound, Ethan believes most of what makes one cannabis plant different from another comes down to what it smells like.

If you've ever flipped through a copy of *High Times*, you've likely encountered those pot-porn centerfolds where a cosmetically appealing cannabis flower is photographed close up, revealing an army

----

* "Chemovar" basically means the chemical makeup of a plant. Ethan never uses the word "strain," as there's no consistency from store to store, or state to state, on the biological makeup of each strain, rendering the term nearly meaningless. "Bacteria and viruses have strains," he says. "Plants do not."

of tiny dewdrops across the plant surface. These are known as "terpenes," which are like essential oils with aromatherapy properties. There are dozens of different types of terpenes (found in many plants other than cannabis), which influence our minds and bodies in different ways and modulate the effects of cannabinoids like THC or CBD.

When Ethan mentions "myrcene," he's referencing a terpene found in hops and lemongrass, as well as in cannabis, that delivers a sedated, pain-relieving effect—which is great for exercise recovery but not so much when doing cardio.

"For clarity and wakefulness you want the terpene alpha-pinene," Ethan tells me. "This can reduce or eliminate the short-term memory impairment THC produces. Limonene is a great mood enhancer when combined with THC, and can enhance the enjoyment of a lot of activities. In a situation where a sport presents a danger, you don't want very much THC. You want a terpene with an antianxiety effect like linalool. The terpene caryophyllene doesn't have any psychoactive effect, but it is a strong anti-inflammatory with some painkilling properties, which could give an endurance athlete that extra push they need after they've been at it awhile."

At this point, many of you are probably wondering the same thing I am: This information is all well and good for a scientist, but how the hell do I apply this to my cannabis routine? If you live in a black market state, the only thing on the menu is likely just "weed," with most of the terpenes crushed and extinguished when it was smuggled across the border inside the rolling tire of a pickup truck.* In my experience, even most dispensary budtenders don't have a clue

....

* For any illegal growers reading this who take pride in the quality of their product and are offended by this characterization, I apologize. Admittedly, I haven't consumed black market cannabis in many years, not since my days selling bricked schwag in Iowa.

about the various terpenes in the flower they're selling, and are relegated to "indica" or "sativa" as their only descriptors—two botanical terms that have been etymologically bastardized by marketing campaigns to the point where they have no relation to their original meaning. And when it comes to edibles, your choices are mostly differentiated only by flavor—which is absurd, considering you taste it for a few seconds but feel the effect for several hours.

"What you need is a certificate of analysis available for each particular chemovar and a book you could flip through showing you all the different combinations of terpenes and cannabinoids you want," he says. "It's possible to do, but unless there's a mandate for companies to provide this to the customers, they're not going to voluntarily spend the money on it. Also, government regulators could require this."

I want to ask Ethan more about this, but the athletics panel is beginning, and I zip my mouth shut.

In her opening statement, cannabis researcher and panel moderator Dr. Sue Sisley goes right for the jugular by saying, "Isn't it interesting that the pro sports with the high proportion of white people, like Major League Baseball and the National Hockey League, have the most lenient penalties for cannabis consumption, while those of predominantly Black people, like the National Football League and National Basketball Association, have the harshest?"

As of fall 2019, this is certainly true.

The 7.5 percent Black Major League Baseball has a reputation for not testing its players for cannabis very often, and when it does, the penalties are often minor. (Unless you're Brewers pitcher Jeremy Jeffress, who narrowly avoided losing his career for treating his epilepsy with cannabis. Though Jeffress is also Black, so Sue Sisley's point still stands.)

"The NHL has really turned a blind eye to THC," says former

Philadelphia Flyers enforcer and panel member Riley Cote, who admits he was consuming cannabis all through his career and now has his own cannabis line for athletes called BodyChek Wellness.*

This is markedly different from the NBA and NFL, which are 74 percent and 70 percent Black, respectively.

Heisman Trophy winner Ricky Williams was derailed from his career with the Dolphins because of a positive drug test for cannabis. Cowboys defensive end Randy Gregory went from a number one draft pick to the second round because of a dirty urinalysis, and was repeatedly suspended for a straight 616 days after a series of repeated failed drug tests. Laremy Tunsil is believed to have lost $10 million on his rookie NFL contract when he went from a projected number one draft pick to number thirteen after a video of him smoking out of a gas mask (sigh) dropped minutes before the draft began.

Colts punter Pat McAfee only tweeted out a happy 420 to his followers—while clearly stating that he does not partake—and was quickly slapped with a drug test the next morning.

The NBA is arguably even worse.

A first offense for marijuana use by a player results in mandatory drug treatment, a second in a $25,000 fine, and a third in a five-game suspension, with five more for each subsequent violation. NBA All-Star Cliff Robinson received several of these suspensions for his multiple cannabis-possession arrests, one of which resulted in ten cops pointing their guns at him while he laid on the ground in Portland. The audience gasps as Robinson, a member of the "Athletes for Cannabis" panel, recounts this tale.

....

* Like Ethan Russo, Riley Cote is a big proponent of microdosing THC and emphasizing other cannabinoids and terpenes of the cannabis plant for a less-disorienting, more dialed-in experience.

A similarly terrifying event befell Super Bowl champion Bashaud Breeland when he was held at gunpoint by South Carolina police before being arrested for possession of a few grams of cannabis.

Both leagues have found themselves in the crosshairs of a social justice movement demanding an end to unnecessary police violence and the profiling of Black people. While I attend this panel in 2019, only three NFL players are taking a knee during the national anthem, but in the year ahead they will be joined by dozens of others, and entire NBA teams will boycott their own games in solidarity with Black Lives Matter protests.

And then everything will change.

Throughout 2020, many team owners, managers, and league officials will perform a whiplash 180 on their racial justice positions as well as their cannabis policies. After dismissing CBD pain treatment as simply "hype" in January 2020, the NFL by March will agree to raise the acceptable limit of THC in a player's system by 400 percent, and will agree to test players only two weeks out of the year. And if a player is caught with a dirty urinalysis, there will be no game suspension. This dramatic policy shift will lead former Patriots tight end Rob Gronkowski to announce the end of his retirement, now that he will be allowed to use CBD products without worry.

The NFL will even go so far as to launch a commission to study marijuana as a potential treatment for pain. (The Ultimate Fighting Championship has also partnered with a cannabis company on a similar trial.)

When NBA players return to the game in 2020, they won't even be tested for cannabis, following pressure from former players like Al Harrington and J. R. Smith and coaches like Don Nelson (who reportedly grows his own cannabis and often partakes with Willie Nelson).

These changes in pro sports have slowly progressed alongside national cannabis legalization over the last decade. In 2013, WADA raised the threshold for cannabis in an athlete's system to 150 nanograms, which allowed athletes to confidently imbibe during their training, knowing they could easily get down to that number by game day.

While the NCAA will also increase its cannabis testing threshold, in 2020 it will hold up a bill seeking to allow college athletes (who are not paid) to be sponsored by outside businesses, for fear that players may be sponsored by marijuana companies. MLB will have the same concerns when it loosens its stance on cannabis in spring 2020, allowing players to use as much as they want as long as they're not high at work, and also are never sponsored by a cannabis company.

Until non-retired athletes are allowed to be sponsored by marijuana brands or the games themselves are (CBS killed a medical marijuana ad slated to premiere at the 2019 Super Bowl), I don't think we're going to see the tipping point that Jeff Konin referred to.

Though at the moment, in 2019, a lot of promising developments are in store for us in the months ahead.

THE DOPE SHOW

Once the panel is finished, I walk across the street to visit a dispensary.

Armed with Ethan Russo's esoteric terms like "chemovars" and "linalool," I'm curious to test the budtender's knowledge of plants and products (a semi-dick move, but my curiosity must be appeased). Once inside, I'm greeted by a giant display from the cannabis brand Floyd's of Leadville, which causes me to smile. Founded by disgraced Tour de France "winner" Floyd Landis, it's another one of the numerous marijuana companies selling pain-relieving products under the banner of a famous athlete.

The curious difference here is that Floyd Landis was busted for doping.

Not only did he confess to using steroids throughout his cycling career, but he was also the whistleblower who took down his own teammate and universally beloved sports icon Lance Armstrong.

Having never cared about the validity of athletic competition, I wasn't that bothered by the news that Armstrong had been doping all these years (though it seems that he did destroy a lot of lives in the process). As a longtime fan of Morrissey, Louis C.K., and Michael Jackson, I know what it feels like when your heroes let you down, but I've never had any idols who would be scandalized by drug use. As an outsider, I've always been perplexed when the sports world is turned upside down by doping scandals. It's such a different sensibility from the world I inhabit. I mean, no one really cared when Lee Child revealed he'd been smoking weed while writing the hundred-million-selling Jack Reacher novels. I can't imagine Margaret Atwood getting bumped off the top of the New York Times bestseller list by Child and then complaining that he cheated by using cannabis and that she should be declared the official winner.

The creative world has never been concerned about such things.

No one clutched their pearls in disbelief and demanded the Rolling Stones be stripped of their Grammys after learning that Keith Richards had been on heroin when he wrote "Gimme Shelter."

What is it that makes the sports world so different?

Like everything else in this digital age, it may just come down to branding.

"The idea that cannabis is a performance-enhancing substance is laughable, and I should know," Floyd Landis once told me in an interview that was never published. "The anti-doping regulators take some kind of self-righteous point of view, thinking that sports are some kind of pure thing that should be held to a higher standard than everything else. At the end of the day, the Olympics, the NBA—all they care about is protecting their brand, and they perceive marijuana as representing something negative."

While walking out of the dispensary with some edibles,* I'm reflecting on what Floyd Landis told me, wondering why sports regulators would view cannabis as something negative. I'm not naive, I get it; I grew up an evangelical Republican in the nineties, after all. It's just that the image of the lazy, unambitious stoner is such a cartoonish and inaccurate portrayal of most cannabis users, I'm surprised it still holds such influential sway.

This is why I don't talk about weed with my running friends, and don't talk about running with my weed friends (with the few exceptions of my stoned running friends). Despite these two activities going quite well together, the cultures that surround each of them eye the other with an intense level of suspicion.

This is the struggle of cannabis-centric athletic events.

The stoners don't want to hang around athletes, and the athletes don't want to be seen with the stoners. The 420 Games was building some momentum before it was sold to Civilized Games, but CG filed for bankruptcy shortly after the purchase (though founder Jim McAlpine promises to revive the 420 Games in 2021). Cannabis-centric yoga classes are popping up in Denver all the time, but once the novelty wears off, attendance often plummets, and the events quietly disappear (intense regulations like the ones that put Jennessa Lea out of business are also preventing these events from

----

* When I asked the budtender for edibles without myrcene but full of limonene, he stared at me blankly before saying, "We have cheesecake or strawberry."

gaining traction). The jiujitsu league High Rollerz (where fighters share a blunt before sharing the mat, and the winner gets a pound of nugs) has been finding an audience after being featured in a *Vice* documentary—though such a niche event isn't likely to break into the mainstream.

Ultimately, while plenty of athletes get high when they work out, they're not always comfortable publicly identifying with "marijuana culture." This is more than just the specter of losing sponsors or medals; it's the fear of being perceived as Jeff Spicoli, Cheech and Chong, or James Franco in *Pineapple Express*—despite these caricatures rarely existing in real life.

As I walk down the streets of Portland, munching my cheesecake edible, I'm wondering if my perception of the sports world is just as shortsighted. I mean, if I'm going to maintain that using cannabis doesn't say anything more about someone's personality or cultural identity than drinking coffee does, then I have to accept that someone exercising—or even playing sports—doesn't necessarily mean they're an alpha bro full of rage and homophobia. Even if the culture that surrounds their behavior continues to demonize cannabis.

Thankfully, I'm about to take a break from mulling over this anthropological conundrum and hang out with a bona fide athletic stoner freak.

WERK, NOT WORK

"We really need to destroy the stigma that being high, or any kind of altered state, is a bad thing," says Amarett Jans, founder of the *Portlandia*-esque Mary Jane Fonda event series, which blends yoga, HIIT, aerobics, and educational classes with outrageous costumes, a bit of queer culture, and a whole lotta weed. "We're in a time where we're building a new language, a new narrative around cannabis. And exercise."

Surrounded by long, sun-kissed hair, Amarett's face is somehow both joyful and pensive as we sit in a beer garden in Portland's Hawthorne district. She radiates the same mystical-hippie energy I often encounter in Boulder, yet seems to put a lot of thought into her words, her brow furrowing as she attempts to siphon her great frenzy of passion into the narrow construct of language.

After sitting through so many presentations at the conference—which often demonized THC in favor of CBD, and distanced medical cannabis treatments from recreational use (when it comes to mental health, I personally believe recreational *is* medical)—I find it a delight to spend time with someone who understands the fuel of euphoric intoxication.

"Whenever I'm asked about Mary Jane Fonda, or blending cannabis and fitness, I feel this pressure to break down all the scientific research to convince them of its validity. When really, I just want to say that there's a spiritual, soulful essence to cannabis, particularly when you mix it with physical movement. So, it's a *feeling* you get that can't be explained. You just need to come and try it."

The faraway, soulful look in her eyes when she talks about mixing cannabis and exercise reminds me of the movie *Billy Elliot*, where the working-class English boy auditioning for the Royal Ballet School is asked how he feels when dancing. "I sort of disappear," he says. "I can feel a change in me whole body. I have this fire in me body. I'm just there, flying, like a bird, like electricity." I'm very disappointed that Mary Jane Fonda's annual event isn't happening while I'm in town, because what Amarett is describing comes closer to encapsulating my feelings about cannabis fitness than anything I've encountered on this journey.

For both of us, the experience was born out of the dance floor.

"I was throwing these wild dance parties that would go into the next morning, which was beginning to get exhausting," Amarett says, telling me the MFJ origin story. "I was having so much fun, but it wasn't sustainable. I wondered if I could create an event that would have all the aspects of a party, but people would leave feeling good, and like they'd been productive. And dancing is my sport, so I wanted an athletic event that reflected that."

As with most people I've spoken with for this book, Amarett wasn't introduced to the idea of blending weed and workout by anyone. She'd always been into hiking, swimming, stretching, and aerobics but never cared for marijuana, or the negative image of stoners she'd received growing up as a Jehovah's Witness. All that changed when—at the encouragement of a grower friend, who referred to cannabis as "the green goddess"—she tried seasoning her workouts with it.

"I was surprised how well they went together, and after that I enjoyed cannabis so much more. It felt like the experience was calling my subconscious to the surface, allowing me to get to know my real self, getting to the root of difficult issues that I was now able to fix," Amarett recalls, mirroring the sentiments of PTSD-stricken veteran Brent Connell. "And it was a lot of fun too."

After getting so much out of the experience, Amarett wondered if she could use her party-planning skills to facilitate something similar for others. "I wanted it to be something for every *body*, but not everybody, where it's *werk*, not work," she says, sipping her champagne. "You can't take yourself too seriously at Mary Jane Fonda. You've gotta have some sass. Your most badass, queen attitude. The costumes are more of a vibe than anything, trying to get people away from the typical *Star Trek*–looking workout gear and into something more playful, something with flash, pomp, and attitude—playing with your identity alongside a real heavy beat."

The name Mary Jane Fonda was a clever pun* that influenced the first couple of events—where the attire was mostly leg warmers, big hair, and leotards with skinny belts—but the annual event has since moved beyond the theme of its namesake.

It's also moved beyond just burning calories.

"I've always wanted this to be a mind-body experience. It's a party but with the depth of an all-day workshop. So there's fitness instructors and life coaches. And cannabis, of course."

While Amarett emphasizes that getting high and dressing up like Barbarella before jumping into a HIIT class isn't for everyone—and that a good deal of the participants are on the female/queer spectrum—she adds that "men are invited, but they'll be outnumbered, and they have to hang. They'll have to get dressed up and move their hips. Also, there aren't a lot of fitness-industry people. It's a lot of professionals, like lawyers and doctors and therapists. Really, anyone who appreciates a good beat."

It's so nice to spend time with someone who isn't a scientist or an athlete—just casually drinking an IPA and chatting about cardio-induced mysticism and why there's no good workout gear for weirdos—that I completely lose track of time and am nearly late for my flight back to Denver.

I express my sincere delight in her company, promise to fly out for the next Mary Jane Fonda, settle up my tab, and hop in a Lyft to the airport.

----

* And totally appropriate because—surprise, surprise!—the real Jane Fonda is coming out with her own line of CBD products.

SPIRITED AWAY

On the drive, I check my phone and see a follow-up email from the World Anti-Doping Agency. I'd replied to its earlier message, asking for some clarification on how it determines the "spirit of the sport" and how cannabis fits into this.

This is what WADA sent:

Anti-doping programs seek to preserve what is intrinsically valuable about sport. This intrinsic value is often referred to as "the spirit of sport." It is the essence of Olympism, the pursuit of human excellence through the dedicated perfection of each person's natural talents. It is how we play true. The spirit of sport is the celebration of the human spirit, body and mind, and is reflected in values we find in and through sport, including:

- *Ethics, fair play and honesty*
- *Health*
- *Excellence in performance*
- *Character and education*
- *Fun and joy*
- *Teamwork*
- *Dedication and commitment*
- *Respect for rules and laws*
- *Respect for self and other Participants*
- *Courage*
- *Community and solidarity*

"Well that doesn't tell me shit," I say aloud to my phone, causing the Lyft driver to look in the rearview mirror.

These are the kinds of vague platitudes used by politicians and commencement speakers that have the power to inspire everyone in the room because they never touch on anything specific. No one actively identifies as the kind of person who is against "fun," "health," or "courage." Though some people have their own interpretations of those terms and see them as incompatible with using cannabis.

Before we arrive at the airport, I pull up the 2011 paper WADA put out on cannabis prohibition and discover something I missed the first time around. Buried toward the bottom is a section titled "The Spirit of the Sport," which says that the term is "difficult to define" and "does not rely on established scientific facts."

It repeats a lot of the same hokey, Eisenhower rhetoric of "excellence" and "teamwork," but it's the closing of this section that brings a little clarity to the conflict WADA sees in allowing athletes to use cannabis.

> The consumption of cannabis and other illegal drugs contradicts fundamental aspects of the spirit of sport criterion. The international anti-doping community believes that the role model of athletes in modern society is intrinsically incompatible with use or abuse of cannabis. . . . Use of illicit drugs that are harmful to health and that may have performance-enhancing properties is not consistent with the athlete as a role model for young people around the world.

Bingo. It's not that cannabis offers one athlete an unfair advantage over another; it's that kids may get the wrong idea. The right idea, as my understanding of this statement implies, was articulated most succinctly by former attorney general Jeff Sessions when he opposed legalization efforts by saying, "Good people do not smoke marijuana."

Apparently, kids view sports stars as role models (I say "apparently" because I have spent little time with either kids or sports stars, and spent my own childhood obsessed with Madonna), and so if they learned that these people used cannabis, they'd either have to change the way they think about pot or the way they think about sports celebrities—which, ultimately, would threaten the industry's bottom line.

This makes me think of the iconic Nike ad starring Charles Barkley in 1990, where he said, "I am not a role model. . . . Just because I dunk a basketball doesn't mean I should raise your kids."

This makes sense beyond the right-to-privacy argument made by celebrities. Idolizing sports stars, to me, is insane. Being a professional athlete—or even an amateur ultramarathon runner—requires a level of physical abuse that stretches far beyond what's healthy. The autobiography of ultrarunner David Goggins almost reads as a kind of masochistic snuff porn, where, in the course of his running career, he regularly encounters kidney failure and blood in his urine, and runs on broken legs held together with duct tape.

Honestly, it reads a lot like the autobiography of Keith Richards.

Personally, I've always viewed long-distance running as a hedonistic indulgence that comes with more than a bit of self-harm—no different than a drinking or drug binge. Both will make you hallucinate; both blur the lines between pleasure and pain; and both leave you dehydrated with muscle cramps the next morning.

In this way, it makes as much sense for Amy Winehouse or Lil Wayne to be considered a role model to children as much as any ultrarunner.

"Extreme endurance sports are not good for you," wheelchair athlete André Kajlich told me back in California. "I'm okay with that. Smoking a joint may not be the best thing for your lungs either. In both cases, moderate doses can be good for you, but in endurance sports there's no such thing as moderation."

Given his inspiring story, André often finds himself in the "role model" dynamic with kids—a position he embraces, having authored a children's book. But this can make some parents uncomfortable when they learn he openly uses cannabis.

Not having kids, I have no opinion on the matter (outside of its impact on my right to get high whenever and wherever I want). If a bunch of Phyllis Schlafly sycophants want to brand me a poor role model for children, I'm not going to lose any sleep over it.

Though it does strike a raw nerve in me whenever someone's character is attacked on the basis of their cannabis use—because there's often a lot more to this than just labeling someone a pothead.

To peel back the curtain of the war on drugs is to reveal an industry of racism and classism disguised as wholesome family values. It's a personal matter for me, not only because I come from the working-class, welfare-funded underbelly that was devastated by the war on drugs (though admittedly not nearly as much as Black Americans or the dozens of foreign countries our drug policies ravaged), but also because during my sober, evangelical teens, I actually embodied all the characteristics of the "lazy stoner" archetype—unmotivated, sedentary, depressed.

Ironically, it was the discovery of cannabis at the age of nineteen that gave me my intellectual ambition—and my love of exercise.

THIS IS YOUR BRAIN ON DRUGS

SELLING THE "LAZY STONER" TO AMERICA

All of us are criminals. All of us violate the law at some point in our lives. In fact, if the worst thing you have ever done is speed ten miles over the speed limit on the freeway, you have put yourself and others at more risk of harm than someone smoking marijuana in the privacy of his or her living room. Yet there are people in the United States serving life sentences for first-time drug offenses, something virtually unheard of anywhere else in the world.

—Michelle Alexander, *The New Jim Crow: Mass Incarceration in the Age of Colorblindness*

RAPTURE AND RITALIN

I was humiliated when asked to take my first drug test.

Throughout my twenties this would become a routine procedure, as no factory or construction site would hire you without one. Though shuffling my teenage feet through the hall of that clinic in 1997, head down, cold sweat on my forehead, desperate to not be recognized by anyone from church, I felt wildly indignant.

Drugs were for losers.

Or at least that's what I'd been told by Kermit the Frog, Bugs Bunny, Garfield, and others in the anti-drug PSA *Cartoon All-Stars to the Rescue*, which was screened in my public school and countless others in 1990. Around that same time, a police officer from D.A.R.E. (Drug Abuse Resistance Education) had also visited our school, showing us a display case of various drugs while explaining that these substances had the power to transform us into dangerous beasts who would steal, rape, or murder anyone who came between us and our next fix.

Those with dreams of becoming an athlete, a dancer, a fireman, or of any other lofty pursuit, were asked to raise their hands. Well, you can just forget about that if you mess with drugs, we were told. Particularly marijuana, because people on marijuana don't care about anything, and certainly can't *do* anything.

This dovetailed with the rhetoric I was getting from the many evangelical Sunday services, camps, conventions, Christian rock concerts, and youth groups I was attending at the time (which came to around nine church activities a week). Angels and demons warred for our souls in the invisible, supernatural realm that surrounds us, it was explained to me, and drugs like marijuana opened our minds to satanic influence—and possibly our souls to demonic possession.

I was more bought in on this idea than anyone (including my friends and parents), and so the idea that I needed to be drug-tested felt outrageous. I'd watched the egg sizzling in the frying pan; I knew what drugs did to your brain. Only idiots (like those D&D metalheads who surely had Satan in their hearts) did drugs, and to be lumped in with them filled me with self-loathing.

It was bad enough that everyone knew my family was poor and on welfare; which, in Christian-right culture, was often shorthand for "lazy druggie."

Though in defense of whoever requested I be drug-tested (a teacher, my mom, I don't know), at fourteen I was behaving exactly like the stereotypical drug addict. My behavior was completely un-predictable, often swinging from fits of rage into a catatonic silence. I had no friends, didn't participate in any sports or clubs (outside of church), and, worst of all, I was flunking *every single class.*

None of this was born out of any nihilistic rebellion.

I wanted to do well in school, if for no other reason than to preach the Good News of Christ. At every church event I attended in the nineties, I was told that the world would likely end soon—possibly due to Y2K. The events foretold in the book of Revelation were un-folding on the evening news, and there was only so much time left to save as many souls as we could from eternal torture. (If any of this sounds like some fringe, redneck snake-handling shit, the pulp novel series Left Behind is a note-for-note telling of this theology and sold eighty million copies—along with two film adaptations, one of them starring Nicolas Cage.) My entire life was based around witnessing lost souls, so how could they think I was on drugs?

Well, looking back, hyper-religiosity is a common symptom of amphetamine psychosis—and in late-1990s Iowa, meth was more popular than funnel cake.

In those years, I moved back and forth between public and private Christian schools, but meth use was consistent at both. The anti-drug propaganda we were inundated with was in response to the scourge of drug addiction sweeping the Midwest. And while we didn't understand the social dynamics of the war on drugs—or how the devastation of Iowa's agriculture economy led to a spike in substance abuse—we knew drugs were bad.

At least, the "bad drugs" sold by "bad people."

To combat my failure in school, I was given Ritalin and later Adderall.

The diagnosis of attention deficit disorder and the treatment of stimulants were exploding in popularity at the time (the name Adderall literally comes from "ADD for All"). While it helped many kids focus, it had the opposite effect on me. The only thing it did was speed up the apocalyptic imagery flashing behind my eyes all day, the ominous conviction that at any moment the seas would boil, the four horsemen of the apocalypse would split the sky, and locusts with the heads of lions would come raining down on us all.

Who had time for algebra when you had the mark of the beast to worry about?

Randomly throughout the day, a surge of inexplicable urgency would shoot through me—a feeling like I'd just been sucked out of a flying plane—and I'd stand up, shouting, "I have to go!"

But I didn't have anywhere to go.

Looking back, I wondered how I'd have felt if I'd known that the medical term for Adderall is "amphetamine sulfate" and that, chemically, it's nearly identical to meth. Could I have understood that what I was experiencing were amphetamine-induced panic attacks and not the calling of Gabriel's horn? What would I have done with the information that the makers of "good drugs" were behind a lot of the "bad drug" propaganda I was inundated with? Would I have understood that those railing against marijuana have used racism and classism to demonize this God-given plant that threatens their economic bottom line?

Probably not.

At that time, I just wanted my heartbeat to slow down, and to find a safe place to hide.

REEFER MADNESS

If cannabis has an energizing effect on the brain and body, how did we end up with the couch-locked, junk-food-eating, lazy-stoner-who-can't-find-their-car stereotype?

I mean, it almost seems as if someone made it up.

The answer to that question begins with an ambitious racist looking for some job security. In 1930, when Harry Anslinger was appointed the first head of the Federal Bureau of Narcotics known as the FBN, which later became the DEA, most Americans were not terribly afraid of drugs. However, they were remarkably susceptible to racism, presenting Anslinger with the opportunity to demonize opium via the Chinese immigrants and heroin via Black jazz musicians, thereby ginning up tax dollars for the FBN—not an easy feat during the Depression.

"The Negro population . . . accounts for 10 percent of the total population, but 60 percent of the addicts," he said at the time, pulling the statistic out of his ass.

While heroin and opium weren't a large enough problem to get Anslinger the funding he was accustomed to during his years enforcing prohibition, there was a new smokable plant popping up throughout jazz clubs and in bars frequented by Mexican laborers:

cannabis. Actually, it wasn't new. The plant had been grown in the United States since the seventeenth century and had been a staple of pharmacies for generations. In fact, years earlier Anslinger himself publicly declared cannabis to be harmless.

He was able to divert the public from these facts by ditching its botanical name and calling it "marihuana," a rarely used term that sounded exotic and insidious (i.e., Mexican) enough to frighten the public into associating it with all their worst fears about nonwhites.*

In 1936, Anslinger proclaimed that 50 percent of all US violent crimes in areas populated by "Mexicans, Greeks, Turks, Filipinos, Spaniards, Latin Americans and Negros, may be traced to the use of marijuana."

"By the tons it is coming into this country—the deadly, dreadful poison that racks and tears not only the body, but the very heart and soul of every human being who once becomes a slave to it in any of its cruel and devastating forms," Anslinger said. "Marihuana is a shortcut to the insane asylum. Smoke marihuana cigarettes for a month and what was once your brain will be nothing but a storehouse of horrid specters."

Media mogul and inspiration for the film *Citizen Kane*, William Randolph Hearst promoted Anslinger's theories and stoked racist fears about "marihuana" in his papers. "Reefer makes darkies think they're as good as white men," trumpeted one such article—adding that, under the influence of cannabis, these Black men would seduce white women.

Or, even worse, "marihuana causes white women to seek sexual relations with negroes!" Anslinger proclaimed.

He would plant these stories in the press, then cite the articles as evidence of his rhetoric's legitimacy, thereby creating an echo

....

* There is a growing movement within the cannabis world to ditch the m-word due to its racist origins.

chamber that grew so loud that US legislators were convinced to vote in favor of a federal ban against "marihuana" in 1937—despite never hearing a minute of medical evidence justifying the measure— laying the foundation for the nearly century-long war on drugs.

Anslinger would often drift back and forth between the contradictory ideas that on the one hand, "marihuana" turned users into violent, sex-crazed maniacs with superhuman strength, and on the other hand it could turn susceptible youths into listless, mindless, unambitious zombies. The former worked when playing on the racist myth of sex-crazed Black men attacking innocent white women, and the latter when targeting the influx of lazy Mexican immigrants coming for white men's jobs,* or the nefarious communist plot to incapacitate Americans via cannabis.

This proved so effective that even when overt racism became socially unacceptable, fearmongering politicians still preyed on Americans' belief in an "other" (whether racially, culturally, or economically different) who was so fundamentally lazy and sinful, all they could think about was stealing your money and corrupting your children while living on government handouts.

DIRTY HIPPIES

"Did we know we were lying about the drugs? Of course we did," John Ehrlichman, adviser to President Nixon, candidly said in a 1994 interview with *Harper's Magazine*. "The Nixon campaign in 1968, and the Nixon White House after that, had two enemies: the antiwar left and Black people. We knew we couldn't make it illegal to be either against the war or Black, but by getting the public to

....

* Well, thank God *that's* over with.

associate the hippies with marijuana and Blacks with heroin, and then criminalize both heavily, we could disrupt those communities. We could arrest their leaders, raid their homes, and vilify them night after night on the evening news."

When conservative Americans viewed the counterculture movement of the sixties and seventies on the evening news, they didn't see an artistic revolution based on community and spiritual enlightenment—they saw lazy parasites looking for a handout. This was not helped by their ubiquitous catchphrase, created by acid guru Timothy Leary: "Turn on, tune in, drop out."

Intended to inspire youth to rethink the competitive rat race and create their own individualistic path forward (a very American concept, at its heart), it was interpreted by Nixon and his supporters as "Don't work, smoke pot."

While today we associate the sixties with hippies and civil rights marches, it's easy to forget how wildly popular Nixon was (his 1972 victory was one of the biggest landslides in election history, winning forty-nine of fifty states), and how galvanizing the fear of Blacks and hippies was to his supporters.

Country music star Merle Haggard penned a series of counter-counterculture anthems for this movement, with lyrics like "We don't smoke marijuana in Muskogee" and "I ain't never been on welfare, 'n' that's one place I won't be, I'll be working."

In 1969 Nixon coined the phrase "war on drugs" during a press conference announcing the Controlled Substances Act, which dramatically increased penalties for drug offenders and declared cannabis a Schedule I substance (alongside heroin) as having "no medical value and a high potential for abuse."

Seeking justification for this move, Nixon appointed the National Commission on Marihuana and Drug Abuse, tasked with investigating the social and medical science surrounding the plant. When the commission returned to Congress with a report titled "Marihuana: A Signal of Misunderstanding," arguing that cannabis is not harmful, doesn't present a threat to society, and should be decriminalized, it was vilified and buried.

Seeking a counterpoint, southern senator James Eastland launched the Senate subcommittee hearings titled "Marihuana-Hashish Epidemic and Its Impact on United States Security." Known as the godfather of Mississippi politics, who once declared African Americans "an inferior race" and the civil rights movement as promoting "the mongrelization of the white race," Senator Eastland was the ideal torchbearer for Nixon's strategy of disarming hippies and Blacks via drug laws.

Hearing only from those with a negative view of marijuana—who claimed the plant caused brain damage, impotence, obesity, impaired immune function, uncontrollable homosexuality, and breast development among men, and, of course, laziness—Eastland proudly declared, "We make no apology for the one-sided nature of our hearings—they were deliberately planned that way."

The hearing leaned heavily on the condition of "amotivational syndrome," which was said to be a state of stupefied, zombielike behavior on the part of marijuana users, which explained the "dropout" mentality of hippies and poor people on welfare.

Inspired by the Eastland hearings, the newly minted National Institute on Drug Abuse gobbled up taxpayer funds for studies looking for a scientific basis for amotivational syndrome. In one study, Dr. Robert Heath of Tulane University—known for his unethical "conversion therapy" tests on homosexual men involving electrodes, prostitutes, and legal coercion—strapped gas masks on a team of rhesus monkeys, forcing them to inhale the equivalent of sixty-three joints in five minutes. When the monkeys wound up with brain damage, Heath claimed to have found evidence of cannabis's detrimental effect, and not, as many pointed out, a case of suffocation

and carbon monoxide poisoning. Heath's study was never duplicated, and his experiment was repudiated by the National Center
for Toxicological Research.

The more funding that was shoveled into NIDA to provide scientific evidence of marijuana's evil charms—with the hopes of justifying its prohibition—the more evidence yielded its medical benefits.
In time, the reputations of both Anslinger and Nixon were severely
tarnished, and many were beginning to rethink their approach to
drugs in America. (Years later it would be revealed that Anslinger
had spent the second half of his life addicted to injected morphine,
and Nixon was often so sloshed on Seconal and gin he would miss
important meetings during national crises.)

People often forget that throughout the 1970s a wave of reforms
led to cannabis's being decriminalized in Minnesota, Alaska, Colorado, Maine, New York, North Carolina, Mississippi, and Nebraska.*
For a while, it was even looking like President Jimmy Carter would
federally decriminalize cannabis, which would surely lead to a fully
legal system within a matter of years, thereby undoing a great deal of
Nixon's racist war on drugs.

But then a Hollywood cowboy came to town and turned back
the clock.

WELFARE QUEENS

"Leading medical researchers are coming to the conclusion that
marijuana, pot, grass, whatever you want to call it, is probably the

---

* Though "decriminalization" reduced penalties only for possession, and in some cases
recriminalization initiatives overturned these changes—and without full legalization,
there was no way to legally grow or sell the plant outside the black market.

most dangerous drug in the United States," then–presidential candidate Ronald Reagan said in 1980.

Viewed at the time as the best hope for a conservative revolution since Barry Goldwater, Reagan effectively created the classist (and racist) "welfare queen" trope—characterizing all poor people as unwilling to work because the government will take care of them—with the aim of demonizing social programs like food stamps, mental health care, and housing assistance, while subtly tapping into middle-class bigotry against poor minorities. The not-so-subtle message was that welfare recipients were both sneaky and lazy, mooching off the hardworking "real American" taxpayers—and we must weed them out of the system.

Throughout his career, Reagan effectively dismantled a number of social programs, cut the taxes that funded them, and successfully took on the unions fighting for the rights and wages of working poor people. Though his biggest legacy was to pick up where Anslinger and Nixon left off with the war on drugs.

And he really had it in for weed.

Foreign relations were upturned to accommodate seizures of pot in international waters. South American countries were pressured to spray harmful herbicides on suspected marijuana fields (poisoning the land, water, and human residents). Any positive reference to marijuana was scrubbed from NIDA databases, and any government scientist contradicting the party line was fired. Mandatory minimum sentences forced judges to pass outrageous, decades-long prison terms for minor marijuana infractions, causing an explosion in the prison population. Asset forfeiture created a lucrative revenue source for law enforcement, incentivizing the extrajudicial prosecution of both dealers and users—often creating cases of guilty-until-proven-innocent shakedowns when someone is found with a joint.

Within a generation, this would lead to the United States having the largest prison system—and the nation with the largest amount of its population incarcerated—in the world.

Reagan's victory to the White House has often been credited to the surge of evangelical Christian voters (who'd previously stayed away from politics) suddenly entering the game, thanks to the organizational efforts of doomsday preachers like Pat Robertson and Jerry Falwell. From then on, conservative politicians were incentivized to focus all their efforts on law-and-order, tough-on-crime, family-values legislation (as opposed to the libertarian tradition of limited government and self-determination), often competing with one another to see who could be the most anti-drug, Dirty Harry cop in town.

Around the same time, the president's wife, Nancy, made anti-drug propaganda the center of her role as First Lady. Though unlike Betty Ford and her message of compassion and treatment for addicts, Nancy Reagan wasn't fucking around.

"If you're a casual user [of drugs], you're an accomplice to murder," Nancy Reagan said in her opening remarks during a council on drug abuse. "There is no middle ground."

With this fire in her eyes, she launched the "Just Say No" campaign.

Through TV advertisements, school assemblies, and "hip" music videos, T-shirts, and cartoons, Nancy's campaign was internationally acclaimed and, at least in the mainstream media, universally celebrated. "Just Say No" cited little to no science or experts, and didn't distinguish marijuana from hard drugs like crack or heroin, focusing instead on character assassinations of those who used any drugs and painting them as evil losers to be avoided at all costs.

Operating under the guise of public health, "Just Say No" focused on the criminality of the substances, not their ill effects. Prescription drug abuse, alcoholism, and nicotine addiction, while profoundly more destructive and prevalent than marijuana use, were never a target of Nancy's ire. This could, in part, be because she and Ronald were both drinkers, he'd starred in cigarette advertisements in the past, and she was heavily addicted to prescription tranquilizers, alongside her daughter, Patti, who was pilfering Nancy's stash from the medicine cabinet. (As was Reagan-appointed chief justice of the Supreme Court William Rehnquist, who, during Reagan's first year in office, was hospitalized with tranquilizer psychosis. This did not deter him from approving a forty-year sentence to a man who'd sold a small amount of marijuana.)

"Just Say No" spawned an industry of anti-drug propaganda, creating a highly lucrative, single-brand advertising market where the top ad firms in the nation competed to create the most disturbing— yet wildly simplistic—portrayal of substance abuse the world had ever seen.

It also helped launch an industry of casual drug testing, which would've been seen as a violation of civil liberties in the past but slowly became a customary routine for getting a job, fulfilling probation, or, in many cases, getting welfare.

After launching his career around the idea that both welfare recipients and drug users are lazy and un-American, Reagan made mandatory drug tests for welfare recipients a wildly popular idea in his conservative revolution. His followers were eventually able to see this to fruition with the Personal Responsibility and Work Opportunity Reconciliation Act of 1996, which authorized states to hold a person's benefits until they submitted a clean urinalysis.

A study from ThinkProgress revealed that after seven states had spent more than $1 million drug-testing food stamp recipients, six of the seven had a positive test rate of less than 1 percent (meanwhile, drug use for the population as a whole hovers around 9 percent).

Missouri alone spent $336,000 on drug tests for 38,970 welfare recipients—while discovering only 48 drug users among them.

None of this mattered, though.

By the nineties, conservatives had successfully branded drug users as lazy dopers (hence their need for welfare) and claimed that the best thing for them was to cut their financial aid, make them unemployable, and, if they still refused to stop using drugs, imprison them—often permanently, due to three-strikes laws.

The prison-industrial complex became extremely lucrative for a certain sector of the populous, as did manufacturing drug tests, operating drug treatment centers (which were mandatory with sentencing), and expanding narcotics police squads into military-like forces, whose budgets swelled thanks to asset forfeiture. All these industries had a vested interest in enforcing harsh drug laws and maintaining the public narrative that drug users contribute nothing to society and deserve all the misery that's coming to them.

Or at least the users of "bad" drugs do.

THERE'S NO HOPE WITH DOPE

For generations the standard Madison Avenue advertising strategy was to instill a low-grade fear in an audience—poverty, disease, involuntary celibacy, the humiliation of an unkept home—then immediately offer a solution in the form of some shiny new product. When it came to drugs, however, the mad men who launched the Partnership for a Drug-Free America didn't even have to sell a product, only demonize one (and the makers of this product couldn't even sue for libel!).

The fear was already there.

There was no need to complicate things with data or explain how any of these drugs harmed the brain and body. The word "drugs" did all the work for them. So much so that a single shot of an egg in a frying pan with the tagline "This is your brain on drugs" delivered all the punch they needed. Throw in a celebrity endorsement (or, in this case, celebrity finger-wagging) from morally unimpeachable characters like Bill Cosby or Pee-wee Herman, and suddenly America was hooked on not getting hooked.

This was easy when it came to crack or heroin, and worked for a while with marijuana, but by the late eighties, Americans weren't buying Reagan's characterization of cannabis as "the most dangerous drug in America."

If anything, these stoners looked pretty friendly.

In the 1987 buddy-cop flick *Lethal Weapon*, Danny Glover grounds his daughter for smoking pot in the house. "Why can I have a beer, but I can't smoke a joint?" she whines. "Because at this moment beer is legal, and grass ain't, right or wrong," he explains. She says it's wrong, and Mel Gibson agrees.

The idea that such a progressive sentiment could be found in what is otherwise a war-on-drugs propaganda film illustrates the nation's shifting attitude toward pot. Heroin, crack—those were scary. But a little grass? Come on. Those guys aren't a threat.

So, the Partnership for a Drug-Free America did what advertisers do best: use a perceived negative as a selling point. If the public was increasingly viewing marijuana users as so lethargic they're not a threat to society, then make the lethargy the threat. This was used to brilliant effect in the 1988 black-and-white TV advertisement "Marijuana Can Make Nothing Happen to You Too."

Here we have two schlubby bros in their midthirties smoking a joint in a living room, scoffing at the anti-drug propaganda suggesting cannabis is harmful. "We've been getting high for, what, fifteen years? Nothing's ever happened," one of them giggles while puffing on the world's smallest roach. "Did I get into other drugs and start mugging people? Nah, I didn't do anything."

Off camera, we hear a woman ask if he looked for a job today.

"No, Ma!" he shouts, while nervously stubbing out the roach.

The implication is clear: marijuana makes you an unemployed loser, with the more subtle suggestion that no one will ever want to have sex with you if you're a pothead. The ad played off the Ansingler-era theory that marijuana could be used to sap and impurify any talent, ambition, or sex appeal you had when sober, leaving you a useless parasite on society and your parents.

This tactic has become a cornerstone of the anti-cannabis propaganda industry and can be seen in countless anti-drug PSAs over the last thirty years.

As recently as 2019 the lazy-stoner premise was used in a TV ad funded by Michigan's Department of Health and Human Services titled "Future Self," wherein a slim youngster getting high and playing video games is startled by an apparition of himself in ten years, looking chubby, greasy, and pockmarked. "Don't let a high hold you back," a voice-over commands. Similar to the Partnership ad thirty years earlier, this ad not very subtly pushes the hysteria that marijuana leads to poverty, obesity, and celibacy.

This lazy-stoner trope would, ironically, be parroted by Hollywood in lazy-stoner flicks like *Dude, Where's My Car?* and *Harold & Kumar Go to White Castle*. As much as I've enjoyed Judd Apatow's movies, a few years ago I stopped watching them after realizing they all follow the *exact same formula*: twentysomething stoner repeatedly fails to achieve adult status until some major life event causes them to find ambition and achieve their dreams—which, inevitably, involves giving up weed.

"I hate that you drink so much and that you smoke weed," Bill Hader says to girlfriend Amy Schumer during his ultimatum in

Trainwreck. The message is clear: you can drink moderately, but if you want to grow up and be an ambitious adult with me, the grass has got to go.

FOLLOW THE MONEY

But wait, you might ask, these anti-pot campaigns weren't coming from a company with a product in competition with marijuana—they were merely a collection of concerned citizens laboring in defense of the public good, right? Sure, they may have been misguided, but what profit motive could they have in demonizing cannabis? Well, as Deep Throat said to Woodward and Bernstein, for the answer you simply need to "follow the money."

Despite getting free airtime on major network TV stations like ABC, along with free ad space in publications like the *Washington Post* and the *New York Times*, the Partnership for a Drug-Free America has been spending around a million dollars a day on advertising over the course of multiple decades, according to the *Los Angeles Times*. Since 1985, it has employed 250 of the top advertising agencies in the country, which aggressively compete with one another for the coveted role of selling sobriety.

But even with the generous flow of cash from government agencies, and donations from nervous "Think of the children!" housewives, a stronger, more reliable funding source was required to maintain the round-the-clock propaganda machine convincing Americans to avoid illicit highs.

Enter Big Tobacco, Alcohol, and Pharma.

It should come as no surprise that the profits of companies selling socially acceptable intoxicants were bankrolling efforts to convince kids that potheads were losers. Seeing as marijuana's appeal isn't bound by any age, race, political affiliation, culture, or geography, and has been increasingly considered as a healthy alternative to booze and cigarettes, it's understandable that the purveyors of legal highs would be concerned about the increasing popularity of their cheap, unregulated competitor.

Cannabis has been viewed as a threat to the legal industry of intoxicants ever since the repeal of prohibition in 1933, when distilleries began financing anti-cannabis movies (some written by Harry Anslinger himself) like *Marijuana!* and *Tell Your Children*—better known by its later title, *Reefer Madness*. And for those who wanted to quit smoking tobacco but yearned to smoke *something* at the end of the day, cannabis was a healthier alternative with a more soothing buzz. By the 1990s, Willie Nelson had been publicly proclaiming that switching to weed helped get him off cigarettes and generally improved his life in a number of ways. And when it came to advertisers worried about a celebrity endorsement of their competition's product, Willie Nelson (like cannabis itself) reached the holy grail of demographics: young, old, rich, poor, conservative, liberal . . .

Throughout the eighties and nineties, one of the Partnership's largest sources of funding were alcohol and cigarette companies, both of which had been severely restricted in their advertising capabilities at the time via new federal regulations.

If, having once dominated the advertising industry, Big Tobacco and Alcohol weren't allowed to promote their products in the ways they'd become accustomed, they could at least smear the competing product by defaming its users. For generations, cigarettes had been portrayed in advertising as a sign of sophistication and intelligence, while a beer was something earned after a hard day's labor or to celebrate your popularity at a busy pool party. And a whiskey on the rocks sipped by a dapper man in a tuxedo implied that someone was getting laid tonight.

If you were asked to describe the mirror opposite of these characteristics—unintelligent, immobile, clumsy, lethargic, sexually unappealing—you'd have the exact character described in nearly every anti-pot ad over the last thirty years.

D.A.R.E. was also a recipient of tax-free donations from alcohol and tobacco companies. Founded by LA police chief Daryl Gates (known for his paramilitary approach to law enforcement, particularly around the time of Rodney King and the LA riots), D.A.R.E. brought police officers into schools around the country with the intention of educating students about drug use. Though instead of them grounding their lectures in any empirical data, these speeches were mostly ominous, if vague, morality tales about "bad people" who use drugs.

As someone who sat through a number of these ceremonies, I can attest that participation in D.A.R.E. did nothing to improve my knowledge of drugs—other than revealing how fascinating they were.

But after decades of fighting to keep their advertising away from the curious eyes of children, allowing cigarette and alcohol companies to bankroll the anti-drug campaigns appearing in schools, on TV, and on the radio didn't sit well with the American public. By the end of the century, the Partnership cut ties with Big Tobacco and Alcohol (though its dollars would return when fighting cannabis legalization a few years later), while still resting comfortably in the sedated arms of anti-marijuana's most powerful sugar daddy: Big Pharma.

For someone who grew up in Iowa during the opioid crisis, it is laughable that the producers of OxyContin, Suboxone, and Vicodin are the same people telling the world that cannabis will turn you into a lazy, confused, hopeless addict.

While their conscious efforts to corrupt doctors, get users addicted, and scam a broken health-care system are finally being acknowledged, their decades-long campaign to demonize a far healthier alternative to their products has yet to be fully understood.

The Partnership for a Drug-Free America was able to get off the ground in part by a grant from Johnson & Johnson (makers of Tylenol and other painkillers), and Johnson & Johnson's then–chief executive James E. Burke took control of the Partnership in 1989, shifting the ad campaigns in a considerably darker and more simplistic direction (à la "This is your brain on drugs"). According to a report from *The Nation* in 2014, the Partnership's largest donors include Purdue Pharma, the maker of OxyContin, and Abbott Laboratories, which produces Vicodin.

Eventually, these pharmaceutical companies began to see the writing on the wall and abandoned fighting cannabis reform in favor of just buying up the market. Creators of the Tom Petty– and Prince-killing fentanyl, Insys Therapeutics gained FDA approval to produce the synthetic THC drug dronabinol, and in 2019 the creators of Adderall, Teva Pharmaceuticals, signed a deal with a medical marijuana company to distribute its products in Israeli hospitals (ready to reach the rest of the world, no doubt, as the domino of legalization continues).

As someone who was not only prescribed Adderall as a prepubescent child but also watched my peers move from Adderall to methamphetamine (and then from OxyContin to heroin), while at the same time our childhood pop culture heroes like the Muppet Babies and Teenage Mutant Ninja Turtles were being propagandized in Big Pharma campaigns to demonize a healthier alternative to their toxic products—like cannabis—I am not terribly eager to welcome these companies into the brave new world of legalization.

My friends and family and myself were shamed on a daily basis for our cannabis use by propaganda from the Christian right, the conservative revolution, and pharmaceutical companies, which essentially gaslighted us into thinking that the countless mental, physical, and spiritual benefits we found in cannabis were never real, and that we were all a bunch of lazy stoners who deserved to be in jail.

CH-CH-CH-CHANGES

Despite my being pumped full of amphetamines, my grades never improved.

My panic attacks only worsened, turning the world into a swirling mess of colors, ideas, and information, spinning far too fast for my mind to latch on to anything long enough to complete a single homework assignment. Despite never skipping a day of class, I only had the credits of a sophomore by my senior year and was told by my guidance counselor, "You may as well stop coming here." So I dropped out of high school and, like many friends and family members, went to work at the local Winnebago factory. I still identified as an evangelical conservative, but after Y2K failed to bring about the apocalypse, I began to wonder if maybe some of the things I was taught as a kid weren't true.

One day on my lunch break, a coworker offered me a hit of his joint.

We were driving back from the A&W, slurping our root beer floats and inhaling our bacon cheeseburgers, when he sparked a roach and raised his eyebrows, looking at me with his cheeks puffed out. I was aghast that he was driving while getting high, and my instinct was to call the police. But then the smell triggered a cascade of memories to flash behind my eyes.

All my life I'd been catching this scent, having no idea what it was.

Sometimes it was on skateboarders coming out of an alley, or teens in a parked car blasting Tupac or Korn, but I'd also caught it on adults in church or in the grocery store, upstanding citizens who I'd never thought were using drugs.

"That smells like my dad," I said to myself, ponderously.

While I declined his joint, I did buy one off him and tried it later that night with some friends at my apartment. I can't say I got "high" in the same way I know it today (it's very common for newbies to feel nothing the first three or four times they try weed), though I do recall feeling very cheerful and energized, performing several show tunes from *The Music Man* before my friends sitting on the couch.

"I thought this stuff was supposed to make you tired," one of my friends leaned over and said to another as I was launching into "Ya Got Trouble."

Being high offered me, for the first time in my life, a safe space of authenticity, where my proclivity for intellectual, bombastic rants and glam exhibitionism were something to celebrate, not exhaust myself by keeping them locked inside. The challenges of reading, memorizing, and computing data that had plagued me during my school years suddenly appeared different. They were still difficult, but I no longer viewed these things as necessary obligations, out of reach to a dullard like me. When I was high, the world appeared full of fanciful curiosities—history! science! Bob Dylan!—and suddenly I hungered for as much information as possible, spending all my free time reading, watching documentaries, and listening to every Great Courses audiobook I could get my hands on. I wasn't motivated to impress or appease anyone—or to show all those teachers who dismissed me that they were wrong, that I was special after all—but because learning was suddenly so much fucking fun.

Without this shift in perspective, I would likely never have spent the next five years in libraries, soaking up information like an intellectual junkie. I wouldn't have devoted half of every day to writing short fiction, essays, and exhausting letters to friends, sharpening my epistolary skills for no reason other than the existential hunger to *keep going and get good*. Without cannabis, I'd likely still be a (very bad) employee of Winnebago Industries, dreadfully unhappy and wondering how much longer I had to endure this life before the sweet release of Armageddon.

I also began moving my body every day.

While previously I could spend a good six to ten hours parked in front of the TV, stuffing myself with soda, cookies, and Hamburger Helper, I suddenly found myself magnetized toward nature, spending whole summer days riding my bike down gravel roads, watching the hypnotic cornfields race past in the sunshine. As a teen I'd begged my parents for car rides just a few blocks down the road, but with cannabis, a three- or four-hour walk around town, listening to Frank Sinatra or Scott Walker CDs on my Discman, smiling at strangers and skipping over puddles, became the high point of my day.

And when I moved to Denver and discovered edibles, I upped the ante and began running through parks and across the city, devoting every free minute of my week to the euphoric turbine of the runner's high.

AMBITIOUS STONERS

"Colorado is known for many great things—marijuana should not be one of them," then–Colorado governor John Hickenlooper said in 2014. "Colorado is known for having one of the healthiest populations in the country, and we should not be trying to get people to do more of what is not a healthy thing."

I was in the office of Kayvan Khalatbari when I heard our governor saying this on a nearby TV. We had paused the interview I was doing with Kayvan (a cannabis entrepreneur who went from homelessness to retiring a rich man at the age of thirty-five) so that we could listen to Hickenlooper's concerns about our state's newly legalized recreational marijuana industry, which mostly revolved around the plant making everyone so lazy that our economy and reputation would be devastated by its legalization.*

"Not a single Colorado legislator was in favor of legalization," Kayvan points out,† lighting a joint in the early-evening hours at his downtown Denver office. "And why would they? Craft beer is big business in this state. Hickenlooper made his fortune as a brew pub owner, and that industry contributes heavily to his campaign. They have a lot to lose from legal marijuana."

I'd heard about Kayvan when reporting on Denver's stand-up comedy scene. There was word of a sharp-tongued wunderkind who was using the fortune he made in cannabis to bankroll a number of arts and philanthropic programs, including an underground comedy show where patrons were invited to openly smoke cannabis (public consumption was and remains illegal in Colorado). This was only a few weeks after Colorado's recreational cannabis industry was unleashed but several years after medical marijuana had burst onto the scene, making Kayvan Khalatbari a rich man.

The son of an Iranian immigrant, Kayvan is a thoroughbred Midwesterner. He's a broad-shouldered, truck-driving workhorse who practically lived at his office during those early years of medical marijuana legalization, maintaining a round-the-clock schedule that reflected his Nebraskan work ethic.

....

* Nearly a decade later, and Colorado is more popular, healthy, and economically sound than ever, and Hickenlooper has attempted to become president by touting his successful handling of cannabis legalization.

† While this is nearly true, there were two state legislators who supported it.

As a second-generation immigrant in Lincoln, Nebraska, shortly after the Iranian hostage crisis, Kayvan was an angry loner growing up, and at the age of fifteen hated school and his classmates, despite acing all his classes and ranking as one of the smartest teens in the state.

"I was very stressed and anxious, very bad socially," he recalled to me that day in his office. "But when I discovered marijuana, I found I could be social and do my homework without getting frustrated. It relaxed me and helped me focus."

Following this, Kayvan graduated early at the age of sixteen, moved into his own apartment, and was working as a waiter and low-level pot dealer. In 2004 he moved to Denver, where he found himself caught up in the burgeoning cannabis-legalization movement. "I used to dress up in a chicken suit and follow then-mayor Hickenlooper around, calling him 'Chickenlooper' for refusing to debate whether alcohol was more dangerous than marijuana."

While living in the bed of his truck, Kayvan maxed out his credit cards to launch Sexy Pizza, a modest restaurant that would eventually grow into a successful, employee-owned franchise. In 2009, armed with $4,000 and a half pound of cannabis, he began operating a medical marijuana delivery service called Denver Relief, which would grow into a multimillion-dollar dispensary and consulting company. (To attempt such a venture today would cost at least $10 million just to get off the ground.)

When I asked him why there weren't more ambitious stoners like him, he indignantly replied, "There definitely are—you just don't hear about them as often. But that's changing. We're seeing bankers and politicians and scientists and soccer moms all using cannabis; there isn't a demographic or race or religion that is immune from having this in their culture. It's becoming as commonplace as alcohol."

In 2020 Colorado, this feels like an obvious statement. Today you can be the CEO of a Fortune 500 company and proudly smoke a joint on Joe Rogan's podcast (à la Elon Musk), but in the early days of legalization it was impossible for a respectable person to even speak about marijuana without needing to urgently distance yourself from the plant with a lot of puns and giggles.

Around the same time as my interview with Kayvan, *Meet the Press* host David Gregory held a roundtable discussion on marijuana decriminalization, where he followed up a statement about the increased potency of today's cannabis with, "But I don't really know that much about it."

"When I think of grass, I think of something to walk on," guest of the roundtable Judy Woodruff, of *PBS NewsHour*, added. "When I think of pot, I think of something to put a plant in."

It was odd to me, as a journalist, that seemingly every mainstream reporter tackling the subject was actively attempting to distance themselves from any knowledge of it. A few weeks later, during a live interview with then-governor Hickenlooper at the Aspen Ideas Festival, Katie Couric delivered the standard "I don't know that much about it" line when asking him about potential harms to the state by legalization. At one point she used the term "vape pens" and then stopped herself, saying, "I sound like a druggie!"

"You seem to know a little too much about this," Hickenlooper jabbed.

The stereotype of the lazy stoner was so insidious that journalists across America—whose job is literally to be informed and speak knowledgeably on a topic—were proudly proclaiming their ignorance of the subject they were reporting on. Imagine a war correspondent delivering urgent updates on a pivotal battle, or a political correspondent reporting on election night, following up their coverage with, "But I don't know that much about it." That would be pure insanity. Yet in the early days of legalization, I found myself to be one of the few journalists who could get through a report on the cannabis industry or legalization without peppering it with references to junk food and Cheech and Chong.

A far-reaching study of media portrayals of Colorado's marijuana users in 2013 and 2014 (six months before and after legalization) revealed that "racial, criminal and cultural stereotypes linger in mediated visual portrayals. Relatively few depictions of marijuana users in the US are visuals of ordinary, 'normal' people or families."

The study found that, across the board, images of racial minorities being arrested were portrayed in stories about Colorado's cannabis legalization, along with pop culture images of cannabis users being lazy and confused.

"Broadly," the authors wrote, "this study suggests that 'ready-made' images of what marijuana users are supposed to look like are indeed being used and reinforced by the media. . . . The heavy reliance on stereotypes of marijuana users is an ethical issue, as media representations will influence how audiences draw conclusions about marijuana use, judge the character of its users, and continue to either stigmatize users or open up new spaces within commercial media culture for alternate, more mainstreamed marijuana use."

THE CANNABIS CLOSET

One night in 1969, a man stoned on marijuana was taking a shower with his wife when he realized he could explain the origins of racism with a bell curve. Excited, he drew a graph with the Gaussian distribution curves, along with a few data points, on the shower wall with a bar of soap.

Inundated with new insights, he jumped out of the shower and, naked and dripping with water, began to furiously write at his desk. "One idea led to another," the man recalled, "and at the end of about an hour of extremely hard work I found I had written eleven short essays on a wide range of social, political, philosophical, and human biological topics."

This is the kind of story that would elicit giggles and eye rolls from those who believe pot-induced wisdom is inherently ridiculous. Though anyone would have to sit up and take notice when it's revealed that the naked man was the renowned astrophysicist and host of the popular science TV program *Cosmos*, Carl Sagan, who went on to use much of this writing "in university commencement addresses, public lectures, and in [his] books."

In the 1970s, Sagan was one of the most well-known and respected names in space science. Hence his being tapped to head up the Voyager program, sending a probe into deep space with a series of recorded music and messages imprinted on two gold records that would play for any alien life-form that encountered it (which, looking back, is quite a stoner idea). Few at the time knew that he was a regular and enthusiastic user of cannabis, often encouraging his colleagues to imbibe at parties.

"He was also the hardest-working individual I've ever met," his friend Lester Grinspoon recalled in an interview with *Vice*. "When people try to say that marijuana will make you less productive, or lazy, and so forth, I always think of him. He was constantly working, in a sense. Using marijuana as a creative stimulant."

When Grinspoon encouraged him to contribute an essay to his book *Marihuana Reconsidered* (from which the story above about his shower insights was taken), Sagan had no shortage of praise and anecdotes about his experiences with cannabis but ultimately decided that he couldn't have his name appear next to these confessions in Grinspoon's book, instead deciding to hide behind the byline "Mr. X."

After all, the book was published the same year that Nixon announced his "all-out war on drugs," classifying marijuana as being as dangerous as heroin. "As much as he loved marijuana, he was always very concerned about people finding out," Grinspoon said. "Really, it was very important that he not get in trouble. He was testifying before NASA and Congressional committees all the time."

One can only imagine the impact it would've had if the "hardest working" and most respected astrophysicist in America revealed that he was a stoner.

Throughout the twentieth century, there have been scores of characters just like Sagan, highly regarded members of society who enjoy cannabis in the privacy of their homes (and even experience a boost in intellectual or athletic performance from the herb) but would never risk their careers and reputation by publicly endorsing such behavior.

In 2012 the famed neurologist Oliver Sacks revealed in his book *Hallucinations* that his repeated use of cannabis (along with other psychotropics) had an enormously beneficial impact on him both as a scientist and as a person. Though most of these experiences occurred in the sixties, when Sacks was an unknown medical student, when he recalled these experiences in 2012, Sacks was only a few years from death, and cannabis was becoming legal. If he'd been so vocal about the intellectual benefits of cannabis throughout his career, it's difficult to imagine Robin Williams ever playing him in a movie (as he did in *Awakenings*).

Molecular biologist and discoverer of the double-helix DNA Francis Crick was playing with fire when he added his name to the Beatles infamous advertisement in the *Times of London* calling for a rescheduling of marijuana, though his signature was one of many, and he was endorsing only legal reform. If Crick were proudly waving a smoldering joint down Carnaby Street and admitting he loved pot and LSD (which was true), I don't think he would've had much of a career.

Similarly, it's difficult to imagine Bill Gates or Steve Jobs getting their start-ups bankrolled if they'd made bong rips a central part of their origin story (which would've also been the truth).

Cannabis has been at the center of some of the most brilliant ideas, and been an integral lifestyle accessory for some of the most enchanting minds, in our nation's history. Yet much of this is being discovered only now, as career success in nearly any industry has previously depended on stoners remaining in the closet. The only people exempt from this conundrum have been those with no career ambition—by no means worthless people, but uninterested in socially championed accomplishment.

And so it's only the dropout potheads that society ever sees.

This cultural representation of stoners as incapable of academic, financial, or athletic success was the perfect narrative for anti-cannabis advertisers as well as the purveyors of movies, TV shows, and the nightly news looking for a simplistic archetype to portray cannabis users. Eventually stoners were reduced to the role of a harmless jester, a couch-locked idiot who may unintentionally say something humorous every once in a while but never actually accomplishes anything (à la Brad Pitt in *True Romance*).

This dynamic mirrors that of LGBTQ+ representation throughout the last fifty years. When I was a kid, the only gay men on TV or in movies were flamboyant, effeminate, helplessly prissy, and typically carrying a poodle. This narrow view of a vibrant culture made it easy to demonize the gay "lifestyle," or at the very least compartmentalize it into something wacky and exotic. Though when the fight for same-sex marriage brought real-life gay couples onto the evening news, society was confronted with the diverse reality of LGBTQ+ citizens. They were schlubby, basic, McDonald's-eating,

Walmart-shopping, Crocs-wearing Americans who were often indistinguishable from their heterosexual counterparts.*

We're seeing a similar dynamic unfold today with marijuana.

Ambitious stoners like Kayvan Khalatbari who proudly champion their cannabis use, and the revelation that some of history's greatest minds were stimulated by weed, alongside TV shows like *High Maintenance* and movies like *American Beauty*, are helping rewrite the stoner archetype—or perhaps acknowledging that one has never existed at all. A filmmaker like Jordan Peele can now freely admit that he wrote the screenplay of *Get Out* while high on cannabis, and Kamala Harris can joke about her youth spent smoking joints and listening to 2Pac while running for vice president.

In the following chapter we'll explore the potential harms of excessive cannabis use, which has led to a small minority of ganja gluttons embodying elements of the lazy-stoner archetype, though it's wildly unfair and inaccurate to judge a substance by the small number of people who abuse it. We don't lump anyone who drinks a glass of wine at a wedding with the wet-brained, skid row derelict throwing up on himself in an alley any more than we associate someone enjoying ice cream in the park with the morbidly obese, bed-ridden gourmand who eats ten thousand calories for breakfast.

When it comes to addiction, there has been too much emphasis on the substance itself and never the underlying need for the substance, which is often the root of any lethargy attributed to cannabis use. As famed nutritionist Dr. Andrew Weil once said, "It's amotivation that leads to excessive marijuana use, not the other way around."

....

* I think this freaked out conservatives even more than the San Francisco leather daddies.

IS RUNNING HIGH ADDICTIVE?

AND WHAT DOES THAT EVEN MEAN?

The opposite of addiction isn't sobriety. It's connection. It's all that will help in the end. If you are alone, you cannot escape addiction. If you are loved, you have a chance. For a hundred years we have been singing war songs about addicts. All along, we should have been singing love songs to them.

—Johann Hari, *Chasing the Scream: The First and Last Days of the War on Drugs*

RUNNING UP THAT HILL

It's 2017 and I'm about to run my first trail race.

In the years ahead, trail races will become a central fixture of my year, dictating my training and vacation plans (much to the chagrin of whatever romantic partner had the misfortune of hitching themselves to me at the time). But today it's 2017, and I feel nervously unprepared for the mysteries awaiting me on that mountain peak.

For the most part I've always been a city runner, accustomed to navigating puking drunks, political marches, and distracted drivers, but feel completely lost whenever I'm running on trails.

Top Five Songs for Running in the City:
"In the City," The Jam
"Wild in the Streets," Circle Jerks
"I Love Livin' in the City," Fear
"Living for the City," Stevie Wonder
"Uptown Girl," Billy Joel

Drop me in any city, and I can always orient myself with buildings, public art, and homeless camps and be able to get around. But whenever friends take me to mountain trails, all the greens, browns, and grays bleed together, and I become lost in minutes.

So the Ragnar Relay is quite the culture shock for me.

It's a twenty-four-hour relay race where teams of eight people collectively run 114 miles up and down a mountain over the course of three different runs each. In the pace of the relay there's generally around a four-to-six-hour break for each runner between their races, which is enough time to let your body go into rest-and-repair mode but not enough for a night's sleep (which wouldn't be possible anyway, since each runner ends up racing at some point in the middle of the night).

Compared with serious ultramarathon races, this is bumper bowling. The well-manicured trail is peppered with lights, volunteers, and other runners every two hundred yards or so, making it next to impossible to get lost (yet I somehow manage to more than once). Nothing like the unmarked, bramble-covered trails of the Barkley Marathons in rural Tennessee, or the rocky, 130-degree trail of the Death Valley Marathon, which will melt your shoes down to your feet if you run too slow.

It is 85 degrees when I run my first lap in the afternoon, climbing for three miles while listening to a playlist I made of songs about mountains, before plunging back down.

Top Five Songs for Running in the Mountains:
"Mountain Song," Jane's Addiction
"High on a Mountain Top," Loretta Lynn
"Rocky Mountain High," John Denver
"Big Rock Candy Mountain," Harry McClintock
"Misty Mountain Hop," Led Zeppelin

The fear of failure has inspired in me a calculated, downright militaristic approach to the race. I arrived days early to acclimate to the altitude; planned a regimen of stretching, hydration, and calories; and meticulously curated playlists that matched the BPM of each song to the predicted BPM of my footsteps at various points in the race.

But when I arrive, I'm surprised to find that Ragnar is really just a big party.

This is going to make me sound naive to anyone seasoned in trail-running culture, or even road-race culture, but I am genuinely taken aback by the Bukowski levels of alcohol consumption at Ragnar. Later I will come to understand that this is not isolated to Ragnar but prevalent throughout the athletic world. Beer sponsors are a cornerstone of the running industry, particularly in Colorado. At any given race, there are a number of beer tents for spectators, beer tickets for runners, and a nearly universal conviction that alcohol—or profoundly shitty food—is the ultimate way to celebrate finishing a race.

While there was certainly a time when guzzling fourteen beers and a few whiskey shots before writing a review of the new Jenny Lewis record was not uncommon for me, that kind of drinking had been long since behind me by 2017. I am not here to party. I am here to *run*, goddammit.

Soon I begin to dread the downtime between races.

Long lines extend from beer tents; bottles of Fireball are poured straight into CamelBaks; and jolly, inebriated souls shout, sing, and dance around Bluetooth speakers once the sun goes down. Similar to a music festival, campsites are corralled together in large groups in the valley. From there you can see the headlamps of runners pin-balling the switchbacks alongside the mountain like slow-moving UFOs. Every runner is part of a team in this relay race, mine being sponsored by my favorite bar and vegetarian restaurant in Denver. Everyone on the team works at the restaurant but me (I'm friends with the owner and have spent more time at the bar than any employee, so I'm tagging along for the race).

At thirty-four, I am the senior citizen on the team, and am, in retrospect, probably not much fun.

The combination of youth and restaurant culture inspires a

mighty thirst in my teammates, and after I collapse in my tent following my first race, they stay up into the night drinking tequila
and squealing with laughter. I graciously accept the IPA I'm handed
but give up halfway through it, feeling dehydrated and grumpy.
Even with earplugs, the Saturnalia-like party buzzing all around
me makes sleep impossible. At 2:00 a.m. I sit up, make myself a
peanut butter and banana sandwich, and wander off toward the
starting line.

I have my second race in ninety minutes.

I'd heard there was an outdoor screening of *Rudy* happening
somewhere, and despite a hatred for sports, I'm a sucker for underdog athlete movies.

Top Five Underdog Athlete Movies:
The Bad News Bears
Rocky IV
The Loneliness of the Long Distance Runner
Cool Runnings
Over the Top

I'm looking for the beam of projector lights when an enticing
aroma tickles my nose hairs. Off in the distance of the moonlit valley, a team of runners passes a glass bong around their campsite. One
of them spots me staring, waves me over, and I graciously accept.

The group of three are the same age as my teammates, and while
they are certainly jovial, there's generally a more reverent mood to
the group than the party kids I'm teamed up with. A married couple
named Heather and Antonio DeRose introduce themselves, both
looking filthy and delightfully exhausted from their first runs. A
slim, hyper gal in her midtwenties named Lia Oriel shakes my hand,
saying, "Most people call me Hummingbird." This is due to her

seemingly boundless energy, which is so readily on tap she hardly ever trains for any races. She's just finished her first run, and a plastic bag full of trash she'd picked up while racing sits at her feet.

This is called "plogging."

I'm familiar with it from an *Outside* magazine opinion piece called "Trail Runners Are Lazy Parasites," which charges our kind with being selfish, spring-break party kids who never volunteer to build or maintain trails as often as our equestrian, hiking, or cycling counterparts do. "That's bullshit," Hummingbird says when I tell her about it, speaking as a giant plume of bong smoke escapes her mouth. "Picking up trash is just good trail etiquette—if you're not too drunk to see the trail, that is."

I notice no one around the campfire is holding a beer.

"You all not drinking?" I ask.

They shake their heads.

"Not anymore," says Antonio. He has the slender frame and buzz cut of a newly recruited soldier, yet his youthful appearance betrays a hard-lived gauntlet of twenty-nine years. "I used to drink a fifth of whiskey every day. And I had phases with coke, Vicodin, tramadol, sleeping pills—really, whatever I could get my hands on."

Accepting the enormous bong passed my way, I take a generous hit, asking Antonio a few more probing questions. Growing up around a whole manner of addicts, I have an itchy curiosity for people's drug stories. Like Alfred Kinsey asking strangers about their sexual histories, I often find myself venturing into deeply personal territory when collecting tales of addiction.

"I grew up around a lot of alcoholics," Antonio tells me, the campfire* light flickering in his face. "My mom and a lot of the boyfriends

----

* Readers' note: It has since been pointed out to me that Ragnar does not allow fires at their races, and while I remember there being one, it is likely not a reliable memory. (This

she had. She was always in and out of rehab, and then at home there would be parties, lots of fights. Later on, my mom's medicine cabinet would always be full of pills, which helped with the pain."

"The pain from fighting?" I asked.

"The fights were when I was a kid. The pills came later."

"Did you fight with your mom's boyfriends?"

"Oh yeah. One of them real bad."

"Were you using the drugs to cope with that?"

A knot in the firewood pops, sending sparks into the black sky. Antonio is quiet for a moment, staring at the fire while his wife, Heather, rubs his back.

"I certainly didn't know that at the time," he says, eventually. "But yeah, there was a lot of trauma there, a lot of depression and anxiety."

Antonio's mother continued to struggle with addiction, going in and out of rehab. At sixteen, Antonio was also living a life of chaos that threatened his life and relationships. Heather was his high school sweetheart at the time, but their lives diverged when she went off to college and he went to juvenile hall.

"I was a National Honor Society goody-goody, and wanted to distance myself from anything to do with drugs," she recalls.

After he was released, Antonio had tried to get sober to win Heather back—but as any addict in recovery will tell you, you have to do it for yourself. At the age of eighteen, Antonio was able to quit the coke and pills cold turkey. Over the course of a few years, Antonio reunited with Heather and became the youngest branch manager of a bank in Missouri. (Though while he'd managed to cut out the illicit drugs, booze was still proving too seductive a temptress to shake.)

....

is why eyewitness testimonies in criminal trials are unreliable.) For storytelling purposes, however, let's imagine a fire. A safe, well-contained one.

Heather and Antonio married in 2013 and moved to Denver a little more than a year later. That fact that Colorado had just legalized marijuana was not a coincidence. Heather was a lifelong sufferer of epilepsy, and her doctors had failed to get her seizures down to a manageable level all through her teens, prescribing her medications with undesirable side effects. While she'd dabbled with pot as a teenager, it wasn't until Antonio (as well as veterans she met while working for Veterans United Home Loans) reintroduced her to marijuana in her twenties that she found a medication that reduced the frequency and intensity of her seizures, until they eventually disappeared altogether.

"Before then, I was smoking cigarettes and consuming alcohol and becoming overweight," she recalls. "But when I started using cannabis, I was able to cut out the nicotine and alcohol and eventually start running."

Both Heather and Antonio were looking to ditch their careers in banking and immerse themselves in this newly legalized product that had turned both of their lives around. Looking back, Antonio says he'd often used cannabis to quell his anxiety, but it was ultimately a minor ingredient in the psychotropic stew that was his drug diet. Now that he was only struggling with booze, it had a more pronounced impact on him.

"Once I got involved with the [cannabis] industry and started learning about the plant as a medicine, I realized what it was doing for me physically, and that was when I really started running." As with cannabis, exercise up until this point had been an arduous necessity for Antonio, just something he had to do to help manage his turbulent (trauma-fueled) emotions. But once he learned about the endocannabinoid system, CBD, and anandamide, Antonio thought he'd give mixing weed and running a try.

Like Brent Connell and myself, running high was a game changer for Antonio.

"Suddenly I felt more motivated to run, which was weird, because I *never* enjoyed running before. I had an increased focus and found a meditation in the singularity of running. I often have intensely introspective moments while running high, and can reframe a lot of the traumatic experiences I had as a kid. This led to a lot of understanding about myself and ultimately helped me to give up drinking. It's been four years since I've had a drink, and longer since I've had any drug other than cannabis."

While other pot pioneers were seduced by the more lucrative path of investing in corporate dispensaries producing high-THC products (which dominated the industry at the time), the DeRoses felt compelled to share their story of healing and enlightenment through cannabis. In 2016 they launched Green House Healthy, an educational and advocacy organization touting the health benefits of cannabis that was the sponsor of their Ragnar Team.

I ask them if there has been any pushback toward their spreading the weed and workout gospel.

"Some people are confused by it, but most are just fascinated," the Hummingbird says as she laces up her shoes in preparation for her next run. "I was sponsored by an edible company when running the Moonrun Monteverde marathon in the Costa Rican rain forest—raising money for the Toucan Rescue Ranch—and I couldn't run more than a few minutes without someone asking me about my shirt. They wanted to know all about CBD and pain, but I kept mentioning that running on weed is also a lot of fun."

"Most people here have been cool about it," Heather says. "But it was hard getting the team together, because a lot of runners, even though they consume cannabis daily, don't want to be public about it. But we believe in this enough to put up with that. Beyond the treatment for my epilepsy, I'd never run as hard or had as much fun as when I started incorporating cannabis. Today is actually the first day of my period. Typically I'd be in bed with a hot-water bottle in a lot of pain, but after some edibles I was able to run up the side of a mountain."

Without warning, the Hummingbird sprints off into the darkness.

I take another bong hit, look at my watch, and notice it's 4:00 a.m.

"I gotta race to run too!" I shout excitedly, and everyone cheers like hyenas on ether. I thank them for the weed and conversation and skip in the same direction as the Hummingbird. I am profoundly high as I approach the starting line, barely feeling my shoes tapping the soft dirt. I make it just in time, as a runner from my team stumbles down the trail, looking pale and dehydrated after running several miles with a belly full of tequila.

She hands me the baton and I'm off, hungry for another ass-kicking.

Moonlight reflects off the river that snakes along my trail as Johnny Cash instructs me to "break my rusty cage and run," followed by Jim Morrison asking to "run with me" up the mountain, and David Lee Roth proudly championing "running with the devil."

I easily abandon all thoughts of form and pace and just settle into the present moment, dancing across rolling hills and leaping across babbling streams. The full moon is bright enough for me to turn off my headlamp and let my eyes adjust to the darkness, feeling like some evil panther that just ate too much catnip.

As I enter a canopy of trees, the trail goes dark, and I can feel my imagination warming up. I recall that Ted Bundy briefly lived in these mountains years earlier, hiding out after some brutal killings in Snowmass and again after he'd escaped from the Aspen jail and killed a few more. Rumor has it that many of his victims were abandoned around here, left to rot in the sun and be pecked at by coyotes—their restless souls swimming through the dark, night after night, hungry for justice.

Delightfully scary stories roll through my stoned mind, one after the other, artificially fueling my adrenal glands. Similar to riding roller coasters and eating hot sauce, thinking of scary shit while running a mountain trail in the middle of the night stimulates my evolutionary reward system. It's the giddy thrill of being chased and escaping, over and over again, as each slap of my foot takes me higher and higher (both literally and figuratively).

Top Five Songs to Induce Fear While Running:
"Frankie Teardrop," Suicide
"Hardwired . . . to Self-Destruct," Metallica
"Idioteque," Radiohead (live)
"The Becoming," David Bowie
"Bouncer See Bouncer," Scott Walker

I'm nearly out of breath but am grinning so brightly my teeth become dry. Anandamide rushes through my veins, igniting my mind with pleasure and giving my joints, bones, and muscles the permission to happily crank it up to 11 without fear of pain.

"Running Up That Hill" by Kate Bush comes through my headphones, and I feel a surge of gratitude for this moment, thankful that I live in a time and place where getting high isn't clouded with secrecy, shame, and the threat of arrest but is something to do while racing strangers up a mountain. Still, I can't stop thinking of what Heather said about so many stoner runners being afraid to publicly join the Green House Healthy team for Ragnar—while at the same time this event is chock-full of drunken bros proudly instagramming themselves shotgunning craft beers.

#Ragnar!

How did a plant that holds so many physical, mental, and spiritual benefits (with so few side effects) become a source of shame, while another far more destructive substance became the torchbearing icon of the running world?

The sun begins to peek its head out of the horizon as I ponder this conundrum. The advancing daylight reveals that the steep and rocky trail I'm ascending is actually the spine of a mountain peak. There is now nothing but air on both sides of this trail, and I carefully remove my headphones, taking in the present moment. I've been running at a better-than-expected time and stop briefly to enjoy the view. Snowcapped mountains surround me. Evening crickets bring their symphony to an end as songbirds begin their morning shift.

I pull out my phone, only intending to turn off the music, but then I notice a message from my editor at *Esquire* and make the mistake of opening it. Typically, I loathe interacting with my phone during a run, and am profoundly judgy of anyone with bad phone etiquette, but this was potentially exciting news and . . .

"What the fuck is this bullshit?!" I said aloud to no one.

ADDICTED

The link my editor sent led to *Esquire*'s website, where I see an article titled "'I Was Addicted to Running High, and It Almost Cost Me,' by Josiah Hesse." I was excited to get my first byline in *Esquire*, but this was not the title I was expecting.

It was true I'd written a story about my experiences running under the influence of cannabis, and it was true that it was such a delightful experience that I often found myself using it to soothe the pain of emotional turbulence (perhaps a little excessively, which was my style), and while the word "addicted" had made it into the story, it was mostly a hyperbolic illustration of how regularly I wanted to get out and run.

In the end, any reference to addiction or excessive running was a small part of the article, and was mostly about how addictive exercise can be. Though some senior editor—knowing that addiction horror stories are infectious on social media—changed the headline and even added a PSA at the end, offering links and phone numbers to "anyone struggling with addiction." Suddenly what was supposed to be a fun, Gonzo ride through my wacky running habits became a cautionary tale about drug abuse.

This is the dilemma any drug user faces in being candid about the ups and downs of their chemical lifestyle. Any suggestion of ill effects from overindulgence is taken as a humble plea for help, as though anyone who alters their emotional thermostat is a destitute junkie in need of rescuing. Rarely does anyone have the sober curiosity to view illicit substances in the same context they do socially sanctioned drugs and realize there are sensible and dangerous users in either camp.

For a long time to come, my *Esquire* article would be cited by marijuana prohibitionists on social media, telling me they're praying that one day I'll be free of this affliction. "Admit it," one of them recently tweeted at me, "your life is out of control. What are you at now, two, three joints an hour?"

This accusation seemed laughably excessive to me, as I can't make it through a single joint by myself over the course of a weekend. Still, I am aware of people who will smoke an entire gram of wax in one dab hit (the cannabis equivalent of several whiskey shots at once) first thing in the morning, and, in their case, I do find that problematic. It's an uncomfortable truth . . . but from time to time I do find myself troubled by the volume of cannabis some people consume and feel that those profiting off it are encouraging excessive use with their high-THC products (while ignoring less-psychotropic cannabinoids). When prohibitionists rail about the new recreational marijuana industry focusing its marketing efforts on its heaviest users—just as Big Tobacco did a generation earlier—part of me has to agree that that is happening and that it is problematic.

This is not easy for me to admit, but as a journalist I can't deny it.

I quite often remind myself of the Upton Sinclair line, "It is very difficult to get a man to understand something when his salary depends on his not understanding it." While I strive to hold myself to a set of journalistic principles (Gonzo or otherwise), I can't deny that a portion of my career success is owed to the popularity of cannabis. This reality has the potential to seduce editors and journalists to emphasize the benefits of this substance and downplay the harms, appealing to the pro-cannabis movement with its clicks and subsequent ad revenue. In an attempt to counteract this, I often follow anti-marijuana campaigns on social media, and attend panels where credible scientists explore the dangers of excessive THC consumption.

And, more than a few times, I've judged a fellow stoner's consumption habits as "excessive."

I am aware of the biphasic nature of cannabis, wherein a mild dose delivers energy and euphoria and an excessive one can lead to lethargy and anxiety. I know that for anyone with schizophrenia, cannabis has the potential to exacerbate symptoms. I understand that for those prone to addiction, cannabis can be a tempting emotional salve, which can lead to dependency. And I'm very familiar with cannabinoid hyperemesis syndrome, where prolonged, (wildly) excessive marijuana consumption can lead to cyclical vomiting.

Still, none of this amounts to a turtle fart in a typhoon when compared with the social, physical, and spiritual scourge that alcohol has wrought upon this world.

BOOZE VERSUS BUD

When running the last leg of the Colfax Marathon in 2015, I found myself teased again and again by the promise of the finish line. Multiple times we'd get one or two blocks away from the park, and a sign with the bold, heavenly word "FINISH" would appear in the distance, only to have the race turn left or right, snaking another mile out of our way, bringing the sweet release of collapse just out of reach. Every faculty in my body was in emergency mode by then, desperate to absorb any hydration that came my way.

There were saintly volunteers every mile or two, handing out bananas, oranges, water, and Gatorade to any runner in need. A hootin' and hollerin' dude in a backward cap handed me a cup of what looked like Gatorade. Eagerly snatching it, I tossed it down the hatch, and then instantly regretted it.

Instead of the sweet, thirst-quenching orange flavor I was expecting, I was instead confronted with a warm, flat Miller High Life. Gagging, I looked at the man, who seemed eager to give me a congratulatory high five.

From his perspective, secretly handing me a beer at the 25.5-mile mark was a welcome, charming move that would be greeted warmly by the runners. Whereas from my perspective, he was a prick who deserved a punch in the throat.

While this is a somewhat clichéd observation, I feel obligated to pose the question: What if he were doing this with weed? Not a heroic dose, mind you, just a milligram or two of THC disguised in a sports drink, creating a very mild intoxication equivalent to one beer. Could you *imagine*? Not only would the man find himself in jail within hours, but the race would be shut down and a civic investigation would ensue. Any children who'd attended the event would be instantly raced to the ER, where their stomachs would be pumped and vitals closely monitored.

Every Halloween in Denver we're warned about this very scenario by the local police department, which devotes taxpayer funds to billboards, social media advertisements, and other media campaigns warning parents to be wary of candy that may be laced with pot. Despite such a Halloween-candy scenario *never actually happening*, the sensationalistic hype never ceases to fuel anti-legalization rhetoric.

The only time anything close to this has happened was when two CU Boulder students served pot brownies to their unsuspecting classmates and professor in 2012. They were immediately arrested and charged with felonies. And while this was, admittedly, a total dick move (no one should *ever* be given psychotropic substances involuntarily), the alcohol equivalent of spiking the punch bowl has traditionally been seen as a rascally prank—because everyone knows alcohol is harmless, right? Whereas cannabis is seen as a deadly poison that will turn you into a rapist derelict with just a single dose.

Considering the wild discrepancy in harm, it's a shame that cannabis advocates are constantly forced to compare booze with bud when arguing for legalization. Without fail, every time voters or a legislature is contending with whether to allow adults to legally consume pot, the campaign will recite some of the enormous amount of medical and social science and government committees pointing out that alcohol is far more harmful to humans and dangerous to society than cannabis. Which is really like pointing out an orgasm is preferable to a kick in the face, but apparently it needs to be said. And still, somehow, we currently live in a society that saturates family-friendly events with beer and beer advertising yet is concerned that adults legally consuming a naturally growing herb are somehow a threat to children's safety.

When the issue of Colorado's legalization was brought up during the 2016 GOP presidential debate, former Hewlett-Packard CEO

Carly Fiorina said, "We're misleading young people when we tell them marijuana is like drinking a beer. It's not." In that moment, I, like millions of cannathusiasts around the country, shouted at my TV:

"I agree with you, Carly! Beer is *way* worse!"

According to the Centers for Disease Control, "one in 10 deaths among working-age adults aged 20–64 years are due to excessive alcohol use." And those deaths are skyrocketing. A recent study showed that between 2000 and 2016, alcohol-induced deaths have climbed by 78 percent among men and more than doubled among women. In addition to deaths from drunk driving and sloshed hunting, there is also alcohol-induced liver disease, pancreatitis, and alcohol poisoning. And while it's tragic that forty-four thousand people die from opioids in the United States every year, the number of alcohol-related deaths is more than twice that.

If you're reading this book, it's likely you're already well aware of the fact that there has never been a case of a fatal overdose or terminal disease caused by cannabis use. Plenty of people have taken too much, suffered anxiety attacks, and shown up at the ER certain they were dying, but the many ER physicians I've spoken with have told me some version of "we mostly reassure them they're not dying, and we try to keep them hydrated" before sending them home (a task just as easily accomplished by a friend or neighbor, who won't charge you a year's wages for the privilege). ER visits for excessive alcohol consumption are treated much differently, often involving stomach pumps, resuscitation, and scans for brain damage.

If not a trip to the morgue.

In addition to the hundred thousand lives lost to alcoholism each year, excessive drinking is estimated to cost the US economy around $249 billion annually, according to the CDC. Around fourteen million people in the United States are said to have a drinking problem, a condition with links to suicide, sexual assault, and violence (the latter estimated to cost the criminal justice system $25 billion each year).

And yet . . . is there any other beverage more strongly linked with sporting events than beer? Here in Denver, our baseball team competes in Coors Field, and if you're not enjoying a Coors Light during the game there, you're most likely watching it on a TV in one of the millions of sports bars across the United States where Coors is served. Even watching sports at home you'll still be inundated with beer advertisements at every commercial break, along with boozy billboards in the outfield and commentators proudly announcing that "this game is brought to you by Michelob Ultra!"*

Sports games are known to be a family tradition in many households—and according to WADA, sports stars are role models for children—and it's here that children are exposed to an onslaught of beer branding, grooming them for a near future when they can join the ranks of the fourteen million drunkards in this country. But if some quiet soul happens to swallow a THC edible before walking into that ballpark, or an athlete uses it to recover after the game, they're setting a bad example for—and permanently corrupting— any nearby children, right?

Whenever legalization is on the table, the inevitable Nancy Reagan–era "gateway theory" of cannabis use leading to harder drugs is employed as a kind of trump card for nervous mothers. But researchers at Texas A&M University found that by a wide margin (54 to 14 percent) most teens found their first buzz with alcohol and

....

* In Michelob Ultra's "Get Up" Super Bowl commercial, we're introduced to a dozen athletes rising before dawn to bust out their swimming, CrossFit, and running routines to a soundtrack of James Brown's "Sex Machine," before regrouping with friends later that night to drink the low-calorie Ultra. The unsubtle takeaway of the commercial is that sexy and successful athletes drink our light beer!

not cannabis. And while there is conflicting evidence as to whether teen use of marijuana impacts brain development, there is no question that alcohol has a detrimental effect on young minds—particularly when they start binge drinking at college parties.

Now, let me clarify that I am not a teetotaler.

As I've mentioned, years ago, before I got into running, I drank an Olympic pool's worth of booze every single night, and am grateful that I had a relatively easy time giving that up. I still enjoy one or two IPAs if I'm out to dinner, and even get drunk a few times a year if the occasion warrants it. But I've also witnessed the ravages of alcoholism up close—puking blood, yellow skin, pissing oneself in the gutter, waking up in jail and being told you've been violent with loved ones—with enough friends and family to know that being forced to constantly compare the dangers of cannabis and alcohol is ridiculous.

It makes sense why advocates for legalization do this, though.

When Kayvan Khalatbari, Mason Tvert, and many others banded together to decriminalize marijuana in Denver in 2005, they named their group Safer Alternative for Enjoyable Recreation (SAFER), an acronym intended to convey that marijuana is safer than alcohol. This made an easy target out of then-mayor John Hickenlooper (who made his fortune in alcohol yet was fighting cannabis legalization), as well as appealed to the microbrew culture of Colorado, home of the Great American Beer Festival. When full legalization was put on the ballot in 2012, it was promoted as the "regulate marijuana like alcohol" measure. Without this prism through which to view cannabis ("it's far less harmful than booze, which everyone loves!"), legal weed would've seemed far more mysterious and potentially insidious a venture for many Colorado voters, and the domino of legalization may never have started.

The argument that booze was wreaking havoc on society was, at times, used *against* marijuana legalization. When Howard "Hee-ya!" Dean was running for the Democratic presidential nomination in 2003, he rebuffed a question about legalizing medical marijuana with the argument that "we already have a serious problem with the drugs that are legal, alcohol and tobacco, and adding a third drug . . . is not a good idea."

It's a ludicrous and misleading argument to make, one that completely ignores the nuance of deciding what substances are too harmful for society to responsibly consume and whether the punishments for using banned substances are more destructive than the substances themselves. Dean came to this conclusion sixteen years later, after learning more about the medical benefits of cannabis, as well as listening to his public-defender daughter, who told him about her clients in the Bronx whose lives were derailed by minor marijuana convictions.

"Then it became pretty obvious that poor kids of color with bad educations, they already had two strikes against them and the third was having a joint," Dean said in 2019. "Which after all is probably not as bad as alcohol."

Today, Dean sits on the board of a Canadian marijuana company. Hee-ya!

REPLACEMENT ADDICTION

In the 2019 inspiration-flick *Brittany Runs a Marathon*, an overweight, depressed party girl in New York City grows tired of spiraling through endless nights of booze and regrettable hookups and wants to turn her life around with a little exercise. Her goal of running the New York City Marathon seems laughable at first—when she attempts a jog in Central Park, she's outpaced by walking elementary school kids—but after a few months of consistent running and cross-training, she not only begins to love the strength, confidence, and momentum her new lifestyle provides, but she becomes somewhat emotionally dependent on the practice.

After losing forty-five pounds and getting a slot in the New York City Marathon, Brittany trains excessively and ignores her ankle pain, which results in a stress fracture. When her doctor explains that she must stop running for at least six to eight weeks, Brittany reacts the way any panicking addict would when told their habit is destroying their body: denial. "Just tell me what I have to do to run the marathon," Brittany says, sounding exasperated and annoyed, forcing the doctor to repeat that she *must stop running* until she's given a clean bill of health, which won't happen before the race.

"Next time you gotta listen to your pain," the doctor explains to an indignant Brittany. "You may have done permanent damage."

Unable to handle the withdrawals, Brittany begins drinking again and plummets into humiliating self-destruction, drunkenly fat-shaming an overweight stranger at a dinner party. Once her ankle heals, Brittany is able to get her life back on track, apologizes to the woman she attacked, and eventually runs the marathon.

A similar story befell Wilco frontman Jeff Tweedy.

After years of medicating a panic disorder with cigarettes and Vicodin, Tweedy checked himself into treatment and has remained sober for nearly twenty years. This doesn't mean he has been without his vices, albeit socially acceptable (and even praised!) vices. When *Pitchfork* asked how he was doing in 2007, Tweedy said, "I feel great! It's been three years since I went into the hospital. I've never felt better. I've never been healthier. I haven't had a cigarette in two years. I run four or five miles, four or five times a week. I've been healthy and having a really good time."

When told he should run a marathon, Tweedy confessed, "Well,

I wouldn't be able to survive it. My knees are . . . I mean, I broke both my legs running too much last summer. . . . I had stress fractures in both my tibias from running too much. You know, once you're an addict, you're always an addict, so just because I found something good to do doesn't mean I'm not going to hurt myself doing it."

This is the textbook definition of an addict, someone who engages in harmful behavior and is incapable of stopping despite the negative consequences. Like Brittany, Tweedy likely felt pain in his legs long before the fracture but persisted, likely due to the emotional high—or its just stimulating him out of depression or anxiety—that running provided. In this way, their behavior isn't all that different from Jared Leto shooting heroin into his infected arm in *Requiem for a Dream*, rendering it so diseased the only recourse was amputation.

"Exercise addiction" is not taken very seriously in mainstream society. Much like being a workaholic, overzealous academic, or compulsive philanthropist, being addicted to exercise is often viewed as a humble-brag, like answering the job-interview question "What flaws do you have?" with "I'm a perfectionist."

But as neurologist David J. Linden explains in his book *The Compass of Pleasure: How Our Brains Make Fatty Foods, Orgasm, Exercise, Marijuana, Generosity, Vodka, Learning, and Gambling Feel So Good*: "Many behaviors that we consider virtuous have the similar effects [as vices]. . . . Exercise can activate the pleasure circuit like nicotine or orgasm or food or gambling, and it can become a substrate for addiction as well. . . . Real exercise addicts display all of the hallmarks of substance addicts: tolerance, craving, withdrawal, and the need to exercise 'just to feel normal.' Does this make exercise a virtue, a vice, or a little of both?"

In the world of treatment and recovery, Brittany's and Tweedy's behavior would be considered "replacement addiction." It's like when an ex-smoker replaces a nicotine fix with a sugar rush, or a former drug addict leans heavily into sex and fame (à la Russell Brand), soothing emotional pain with vices for years, and then, when those vices disappear, having some reflexive impulse seek out running as a way to feel the same euphoric charge they once knew.

And they kept punching that button until their bodies collapsed.

This was definitely my experience when I first started running on cannabis, and was ultimately what I was getting at in the *Esquire* story. Throughout my twenties I'd used alcohol and romantic conquest as an emotional salve to nurse the wounds of childhood trauma, and ultimately running high just became a more effective treatment (with fewer hangovers). So I switched. I made the mistake of briefly touching on this in the *Esquire* story when mentioning that, after enduring a particularly painful breakup, I'd pushed myself a little too hard when running in the park one summer day:

> *I'd be dehydrated and malnourished in 100-degree heat, rounding my tenth mile as I cried behind dark sunglasses—egged on by the breakup songs of Rilo Kiley, Belle & Sebastian, and Wilco. If Denver parks had a bartender, I would've been 86'd as an unruly customer.*

This was intended to illustrate how seductive the runner's high experience was though, not that it had plunged my otherwise balanced life into a state of chaos. If I'd known I was writing a story about addiction—as the editor's headline had implied—I'd have mentioned that just because something can be a conduit for addiction doesn't mean it's just as dangerous as any other substance. And just because a substance or behavior stimulates the reward system of the brain doesn't mean that it can't be navigated responsibly.

Generations of Nancy Reagan programming has left our society with a simplistic, binary view of drugs and addiction, endowing all illegal substances with the power to instantly hook and destroy any life they come in contact with, and any market-approved, government-sanctioned drug as free of negative consequences. Rare is the citizen who has a three-dimensional view of drugs, behavior, and addiction that accounts for the myriad ways we all—from the speedball junkie in the alley to the megachurch preacher on his third latte—toy with our brain chemistry throughout the day.

Ultimately, anything that stimulates our evolutionary reward mechanisms has a potential for addiction, and this includes a number of socially acceptable substances and activities. Studies suggest that sugar may be just as addictive as cocaine, and yet we pump children with it at an almost hourly rate. We arbitrarily praise or condemn various pleasures based not on scientific evaluation of risk versus reward but on a prescribed morality that is subject to the shifting winds of time and geography.

From cheese to aspirin to television to orgasms to cocktails, most of us spend our days artificially stimulating our reward circuits over and over like a pinball bouncing between flashing bumpers. Someone will laughingly confess to being a "chocoholic" without acknowledging the emotional soothing they're after when purchasing that rich dessert. Rarely do we take these kinds of addictions seriously (despite disastrous health consequences) because rarely do we see someone contending with the absence of their drug.

For instance, let's imagine a world without caffeine.

Whatever the scenario (let's say an alien invasion steals all the tea, coffee, and Monster Energy in the world), we all wake up tomorrow and the world is rid of caffeine. How many people would be, if not unable to work at all, unable to work very well? The headaches, the short tempers, the depression, the foggy mornings that blend into listless afternoons—a significant portion of our population would become temporarily useless without caffeine, if not suffer complete emotional breakdowns.

Consumed by 90 percent of American adults, caffeine is the only psychotropic drug we casually serve to children (who consume it at a rate of 75 percent, beginning at the age of six), and it's readily available at damn near any establishment that serves liquids. Most of those with a caffeine addiction never become aware of it because they never experience withdrawals. When researching his book *Caffeine*, Michael Pollan took a three-month, cold-turkey sabbatical from his daily tea and coffee regimen, and discovered that in addition to the typical headaches, irritability, and loss of focus and energy to be expected, he also experienced a profound scrambling of his emotions and self-esteem.

"I lost confidence in the whole book. It suddenly seemed like a stupid idea," he told Terry Gross in 2020. "And loss of confidence is a common symptom of caffeine withdrawal."

Wars have been fought over tea for centuries, and coffee has faced nearly as many prohibition laws (and as much racist propaganda) as cannabis. Yet we as a society are far more dependent on it than any other drug. Caffeine is an integral cog in the American machinery, facilitating our productivity, social lives, and emotional equilibrium. Many of us continue using caffeine despite negative consequences, like increased heartbeat, ulcers, nausea, acid reflux, dehydration, mood swings, insomnia, and stained teeth.

Does this mean we should ban coffee?

In my opinion, no.

Personally, I've never believed that society needs ridding of addictive pleasures, but it must acknowledge and treat the underlying emotional pain driving some to self-destruction. If Tweedy, Brittany, or myself are punching the runner's high button so much that it causes our bodies to break down, the runner's high is not to blame, and criminalizing it won't end the problematic behavior. I believe that a sophisticated understanding of drugs and their relationship to our brain chemistry is a more effective tool in combating addiction than jail, social shame, or even sobriety.

When running for sheriff of Aspen County in 1971, "Freak Power" candidate Hunter S. Thompson addressed his plan for decriminalizing marijuana by saying, "Young people have been lied to about marijuana for so long—people saying it makes your brain soft and your feet fall off—it's difficult for them to trust anyone arguing for the prohibition of it."

When examining the number of psychotropic substances Americans use on a daily basis that mirror illicit ones (Adderall is, chemically, nearly identical to meth, as Vicodin is to heroin), it becomes difficult to trust the addiction rhetoric handed down from our government. Or, at the very least, it forces us to contend with the fact that emotional turbulence is an unavoidable part of the human experience, and there are a number of perfectly healthy (and wildly unhealthy) tools to deal with that—with a vast gray area between the two.

GONZO ENNUI

When I first saw Johnny Depp play him in *Fear and Loathing in Las Vegas*, I had no idea that Hunter S. Thompson was a real person. And in many ways, he wasn't.

Like scores of other young (mostly male) writers, Thompson was an inspiration to me. He was a beacon of hedonistic freedom, a mythical trickster whispering in my ear, telling me all the laws of polite society were just made up by long-dead bureaucrats—and I was free to make up my own rules. His passion, lyricism, and boundless courage changed the way I wanted to live my life. The chains of evangelical sobriety fell from my wrists as I followed the good doctor into the sunset.

I moved to Colorado in part because Thompson lived there. But tragically, he shot himself in the head only a few months after I arrived.

For my first few years in Denver, I spent every day at the Tattered Cover Book Store, reading (and rereading) the vast catalog of letters, essays, novels, and reporting Thompson composed in his sixty-seven years. It's often overlooked that before he discovered his unbridled "Gonzo" style, Thompson spent a good fifteen years of his life diligently cranking out straightforward material, and before that spent his teenage years consuming so much literature that one friend said, "By the time he finished high school, he was better read than most Yale graduates."

If Thompson wrote five thousand words a day, so would I.

If Thompson retyped his favorite books, so would I.

If Thompson threatened his editors with violence when his checks were late, so would I. (Note: not all these lessons served me well.)

What a lot of young writers, including myself, failed to recognize is that Thompson could get away with consuming enough drugs to kill a horse* and still crank out decent prose because he had all those years of (relatively) sober writing to build up his muscle memory for facts and sentences. And even then, he was a craftsman of his stories, rewriting *Fear and Loathing in Las Vegas* six times before handing it off to his editor. Whenever any of us attempted to mimic either his writing style or his drug use, the results often appeared

----

* A daily regimen that included a frightening amount of cocaine, acid, cannabis, whiskey, cigarettes, speed, and sleeping pills.

grotesque to anyone forced to witness such a tragedy. But it sure was fun to try this costume on.

I met my first Hunter Thompson sycophant in the summer of 2005.

Jeremy Johnson was a tall, slim guy holding court at a Denver bar, talking loudly and animatedly with his hands. A friend pointed him out to me, saying he was a local journalist I should introduce myself to. His curly blond Afro—held tightly in place with a vintage sweatband—made him look not unlike Will Ferrell in the movie *Semi-Pro*, but with a thick handlebar mustache dripping down the sides of his mouth. My writing career was still in its infancy, and Jeremy Johnson was actually the first professional writer I'd ever met. Like Neal Cassady introducing himself to Kerouac and asking him how to be a writer, I approached Jeremy asking how to make money as a writer.

The closer I got, the stronger the booze fumes emanating from him became.

"You know what a query letter is?" he slurred when I asked for his help.

I admitted that I didn't.

"Well, come back when you do."

Ignoring his dismissal, I complimented the Hunter Thompson tattoo gracing his forearm. It was the Gonzo logo Thompson had created for his campaign for Aspen sheriff, featuring a clenched fist with two thumbs clutching a peyote button. Jeremy looked at his tattoo, then at me.

"What do you know about Hunter Thompson?" he balked.

While I was intimidated to know so little about journalism (having dropped out of high school and never set foot in a college classroom), I had a black belt in Hunter Thompson trivia and quickly rattled off a volume of encyclopedic details.

Jeremy and I quickly bonded over our love of writing and

scrambling our brain chemistry, often closing down the bar before buying a few grams of coke and heading out to an all-night rager in one of Denver's abandoned warehouses (this was long before they were all turned into cannabis grow houses). Our decadent friendship was a short-lived period of my life though, as Jeremy and his blond Afro disappeared only a few months after I was introduced to them.

More than a decade later, I recently ran into Jeremy on a mountain trail just outside Denver. He is still slim and hyper (he's weighed the same 144 pounds since high school), but he's cut his hair short and certainly looks a lot further from death than he did the last time I saw him.

I ask him whatever happened to him all those years ago.

"I had to get out of Denver to kind of clean up my life a bit, so I moved to Pennsylvania," Jeremy recalls. "I was partying so much, and all the booze, cigarettes, and coke were starting to kill me."

Jeremy's relationship was on the rocks at this time, and he knew that his lifestyle was going to land him a wet-brained jailbird, or dead, if he didn't make a major course correction. But Jeremy was also burdened with a terrific lust for life, desperate to squeeze every ounce of pleasure and excitement out of each day—and if he wasn't going to get that via hard-living chaos, he'd need a new thrill to take its place.

Around the same time, my image of Hunter Thompson and his decadent lifestyle was beginning to shift. Beyond my own numerous shaky mornings—staring into a mirror and asking, Is this even fun anymore?—my view of Thompson's character was taking on a new dimension. His life looked like a lot of fun in the books and documentaries, but for those close to him, Thompson could often be a dangerous beast. Reading the memoir of his son, Juan Thompson, I was horrified by the homophobic bullying he laid on his child, but it was also eye-opening to learn of the depression, incontinence, mood swings, psychosis, and financial ruin that came with the Gonzo lifestyle.*

Also, his last few books—while containing moments of brilliance—were mostly as unreadable as the entrails of a chicken.

By my thirties, I'd begun to separate the lessons of Hunter Thompson that were serving me (aggressively follow your passion, work hard, be playful, don't take shit from idiots) from the ones that were dragging me down (cruelty, a lust for fame, the incessant pursuit of euphoric madness). However, with running I was finding that I could still channel that urgency into something weird and wonderful, while still (mostly) protecting myself and everyone around me from complete ruin.

And, it seemed, Jeremy Johnson had been learning the same lessons.

A onetime high school track star, Jeremy attempted to rehabilitate himself via the Oil Creek 100, a challenging ultramarathon through the historic oil country of rural Pennsylvania. Like the Hummingbird, Jeremy was blessed with a naturally high metabolism and VO$_2$ max, allowing him to bounce back into running after a lengthy sabbatical. But while running helped quell his more self-destructive desires, it wasn't until he combined it with cannabis that Jeremy found an outlet for the restless engine of passion roaring inside him.

"The first time I tried running high, it was amazing," Jeremy recalls as we jog down a trail lined with Aspen trees, passing his pen vaporizer back and forth. "I was blown away at how focused I

---

* I had a similar revelation after spending an afternoon drinking and smoking joints with Jeff Dowd, the inspiration behind The Big Lebowski's "Dude" character.

became. People think of pot as some wacky party drug, but that's not the way it is for me. I was dialed in."

We hit a steep, rocky incline on the trail, which demands more oxygen from me than my city lungs can handle. But Jeremy is tackling it with effortless grace, quickly trotting up the hill while talking comfortably, his lanky arms like those of a basketball player ready to catch a side-court pass. It's taking all my mental strength to navigate the rocks and tree roots while also listening to this story, while Jeremy looks as though he could maneuver the whole thing blindfolded.

"My favorite part of running high is the downhills," he says. "Really steep, technical downhills where the trees are buzzing by you and every step counts. It's the one moment in my day where nothing else matters, my head is just completely focused on where my foot is gonna land next. Cannabis helps me find that unconscious rhythm in my arms, legs, and breath that's so essential to good running."

With this kind of intense, Sonic the Hedgehog–style of running, Jeremy was able to exorcise his party demons enough to lead a more stable, balanced life. He married his girlfriend, who gave birth to a baby girl, and the three of them moved back to Colorado, where Jeremy settled into an eight-to-five job at a daily newspaper. It was here that Jeremy began regularly competing in races across the Rocky Mountains, which were close enough to his home in Denver that he could burn off his excess energy on the trails each day after work.

After ranking in the top 10 for his age group for several consecutive years, Jeremy now finds himself garnering respect from those in the running community who would otherwise dismiss stoners as useless. He often weighs in on "running high" debates on various trail-running social media pages (where conservative and hippie runners clash on the topic at least once a week) and replies to those who say stoners are slow and lazy with "Catch me on the downhills and we'll see."

"I don't flaunt it, but I also don't hide it," Jeremy says of his ritualistic edible and/or vape before a run. "People are really weird about it, which kind of bothers me in some ways, because the trail-running community is so interwoven with the craft-brew industry. It's not uncommon to have races that start or end at breweries, or even drink beers on the trails. But those same people get weird if I'm ingesting cannabis, as if it's gonna impair my cognitive abilities and make me a bad runner. It's helped make me the runner that I am."

HARM REDUCTION

Jeremy Johnson credits his ability to quit cigarettes, coke, and binge drinking to his love affair with running high (particularly on trails). And says it's not uncommon for those who regularly run the trails stoned to be in a transitional state of their lives, seeking a pivot away from more self-destructive behavior.

"There's definitely a recovery aspect to running," Jeremy says. "You see a lot of these punk-rock, pirate-type runners who used to live a crazy lifestyle, and this is the way they're gonna live crazy now. Drugs and drinking are ways that some people experience the pain of their lives. And running is also a way to experience pain. So if that's the sting you need to keep feeling alive, it's a hell of a lot better than booze and cigarettes."

If I can briefly contradict something I said earlier in this chapter, I'd like to state that I do not believe all drugs are the same. And perhaps even more important, not all drugs are the same to all people. I know I made a big to-do earlier about how we're all drug addicts of one kind or another, implying a sort of moral relativism when it comes to altering our brain chemistry. And while I maintain that the legal and cultural lines drawn between substances are mostly arbitrary, I do believe that an addict can swap one powerfully destructive drug for a milder, more manageable one as a process of their addiction recovery.

This approach is known as "harm reduction," a controversial form of addiction therapy opposed by those who follow the twelve-step gospel of absolute sobriety. Conceived in the 1970s by medical marijuana icon Dr. Tod Mikuriya, the practice is centered on reducing an addiction down to a manageable level via whatever works (whether methadone, supervised injection sites, or a cannabis replacement program). While some find comfort in the militaristic structure of an AA program, others have found harm reduction a less threatening, more realistic route toward getting their lives together.

Swapping out booze or hard drugs for cannabis makes sense on a medical basis, due to the fact that cannabis is not physically addictive, is known to be an effective treatment for depression, and doesn't cause a spiral trajectory of abuse the same way other substances do.

"People who use cannabis medically for treatment of a stable condition, we don't see dose escalation over time the way you would with opioids, where people develop tolerance to effect and need more and more to see a benefit," says Dr. Ethan Russo. "Often the dose goes down."

According to a study of two thousand opioid-injection addicts attempting to get clean in Vancouver, those who used cannabis had a much higher success rate than those who didn't.

Throughout his life, Dr. Mikuriya aggressively advocated for doctors to be allowed to prescribe cannabis to their patients, turning the notion of medical marijuana from a laughable sketch-comedy premise to a regulated, government-sanctioned mandate spreading across the nation. As his ideas of treating the nausea of cancer and AIDS patients with cannabis grew into mainstream acceptability, so did his theory of harm reduction.

A few years before his death in 2007, Mikuriya published a study in which ninety-two alcoholics found that the introduction of cannabis to their lives greatly reduced or eliminated their alcohol consumption. "Even if [cannabis] use is daily," he wrote, replacing alcohol with cannabis "reduces harm because of its relatively benign side-effect profile." Mikuriya's theory was ratified a few years later when psychiatrists at the University of the West Indies published the study "Transitional Drug Use: Switching from Alcohol Disability to Marijuana Creativity."

"It appears that a marijuana maintenance programme can be utilized in carefully selected individuals as a replacement for alcohol abuse disorders," the researchers concluded. "Transitional drug use to marijuana offers the opportunity of episodic use, less effect on behavior, more personal interest in creativity, absence of bulk and less need for group socialization."

Known today as "Cali sober," the trend of ditching booze for bud has taken hold among those Gen Zers and millennials who have been fortunate enough to come of age in the era of legal weed. Nearly a decade after Colorado legalized it, states with legal marijuana are experiencing tremendous dips in alcohol and opioid abuse (particularly with at-risk groups like veterans and college students).

Though does cannabis have to be viewed as the rebound that follows a breakup and not as a serious contender for a long-term relationship? Does the fact that Antonio DeRose, Jeremy Johnson, and I used running high to transition out of more destructive lifestyles mean that our journey is incomplete until we're as sober as baby monks?

Are we still just helpless addicts?

IS CANNABIS ADDICTIVE?

In 2013, glam-pop superstar Lady Gaga confessed to being addicted to marijuana.

"I have been addicted to it and it's ultimately related to anxiety coping and it's a form of self-medication and I was smoking up to fifteen to twenty marijuana cigarettes a day with no tobacco," she said on *Elvis Duran and the Morning Show.* "Looking back, I do see now that some of it had to do with my hip pain."

Regardless of her intentions, this quote was like catnip to prohibitionists, who pointed to the meat-dress-wearing, avant-garde pop artist as evidence of weed's corrupting influence. When southern senator Jeff Sessions was outraged by a comment President Obama made about cannabis being less harmful than alcohol, he told the Senate Judiciary Committee, "This is just difficult for me to conceive how the president of the United States could make such a statement as that. . . . Lady Gaga is addicted to it, and it's *not* harmless."

To my knowledge, Gaga never made any follow-up comments about her relationship with cannabis. (Though her consistently sparking joints throughout the 2017 documentary *Gaga: Five Foot Two* suggests that she won't be checking into Celebrity Rehab anytime soon.)

According to the National Institute for Drug Abuse, 9 percent of marijuana users develop a dependence to the substance (meaning withdrawal symptoms occur when they try to stop). Which sounds like a lot. Yet 35 percent of caffeine users develop a dependence to that substance, and of those, 44 percent continue to consume caffeine even if their health and life are negatively affected. As you can imagine, the rates of addiction for alcohol (15 percent), heroin (23 percent), and nicotine (32 percent) make cannabis addiction seem much more manageable.

But even those rates of addiction for hard drugs begs some attention.

If only 23 percent of people who use heroin develop a dependency to it, then that means 78 percent of those who shoot (or snort) smack never let it get out of hand. They're able to take it or leave it, never allowing the drug to have a negative impact on their family, jobs, or physical health.

How can that be?

Our "Just Say No" understanding of drugs and addiction suggests that it's the drugs themselves that hijack an otherwise healthy person's brain, rendering them useless in all tasks outside the myopic pursuit of another hit. If only one out of four users becomes addicted to heroin, that would suggest that there are additional (perhaps superseding) factors that determine which camp a user ends up in.

The simplistic view that all drug users are drug addicts, and all addicts are hijacked monsters who care for nothing outside their next fix, comes from years of studying rats pressing levers for drugs or food inside a cage. Often these rats grow to favor heroin, cocaine, or whatever is stimulating their reward system over basic necessities like food and water. Though addiction science is now revealing that when rats are taken out of their cold, isolated cages and placed in a more organically favorable setting—with plenty of sex, toys, community, and exercise—their desire for drugs plummets dramatically.

A similar study—this one on humans—was conducted by Dr. Carl Hart at Columbia University. After growing up around the crack epidemic of the eighties and nineties and absorbing all the government propaganda that came with it, Hart began his career seeking a neurological cure for addiction. But when he completed his study of crack addicts from low-income neighborhoods being offered a hit of medical-grade cocaine now or five dollars at a later date over and over for three weeks, he was surprised to find that subjects would often prefer the cash.

"If you're living in a poor neighborhood deprived of options, there's a certain rationality to keep taking a drug that will give you some temporary pleasure," Dr. Hart said to the *New York Times*. "The key factor is the environment, whether you're talking about humans or rats. The rats that keep pressing the lever for cocaine are the ones who are stressed out because they've been raised in solitary conditions and have no other options. But when you enrich their environment, and give them access to sweets and let them play with other rats, they stop pressing the lever.

"Eighty to 90 percent of people are not negatively affected by drugs, but in the scientific literature nearly 100 percent of the reports are negative," Dr. Hart continued. "There's a skewed focus on pathology. We scientists know that we get more money if we keep telling Congress that we're solving this terrible problem. We've played a less than honorable role in the war on drugs."

When expanding our understanding of addiction, there are more factors to be discussed than just environment—generational trauma and genetic predisposition to addiction come to mind—but I bring up these specific studies to illustrate that our understanding of drugs and addiction is wildly simplistic, and if we're going to take an honest look at cannabis abuse, we need to bring this new information along.

Ultimately, anything that impacts us emotionally is going to have the potential for abuse, regardless of its packaging. The drugs themselves have no moral identity; they are merely tools. And as with any powerful tool, their capacity for harm or healing is determined by the knowledge and intention of their user. A hammer can be used to build a house, or to crack someone's skull.

Drugs are no different.

So, now that all that's said, I will admit that I've known many people with an addiction to cannabis. While this plant is not physically addictive in the same way nicotine, alcohol, and heroin are, there are definite emotional withdrawal symptoms for chronic users—and certainly cases where someone would like to stop but feels incapable. Though now that we've inverted our concept of addiction—understanding that a shitty life leads to drug abuse, not the other way around—we should begin to view compulsive marijuana use as a symptom of a greater disorder and not the cause.

Growing up in an economically destitute, sexually and emotionally repressed, violently cold section of north Iowa, I witnessed that emotional coping via drugs (or religion) was practically a cultural touchstone for my people. When I abandoned straight-edge evangelicalism for Gonzo hedonism, I leaned heavily into booze and drugs as an escape from my bleak existence. It was only years later, after discovering meditation, therapy, and running high, that I was able to process emotions without a chemical fire hose to my brain.

Though my story isn't everyone else's—and neither is yours.

To pretend that we all carry a moral obligation of complete sobriety, and that a universal path toward sobriety exists for everyone, is harmful and naive. If a veteran of war suffers chronic PTSD-induced nightmares and can't go out to a restaurant without having a panic attack, are you really going to say he is undeserving of as much cannabis as he needs to feel better? When I first saw a 600-milligram THC edible on the shelf of a medical dispensary, I wondered, *Who would want to get that high?* But when I began meeting terminal cancer patients and those with debilitating chronic pain—the kind of pain that screams through your body all day and night, turning an otherwise kind soul into a monster—I realized that what "healthy" or "sober" looks like for me doesn't apply to everyone else.

When it comes to health care in America, we have a difficult time swallowing the reality that some conditions do not improve. Regardless of wealth or resources, some illnesses are beyond the reach of modern medicine, and the best you can hope for is stabilization and comfort. This goes for mental as well as physical conditions. And if cannabis can provide some relief to a person without hope, is it really worth it to judge the dose or consistency of their intake?

This includes the junkie, alcoholic, and meth-head on a harm-reduction program. If an otherwise helpless, violent mess can manage to get through the day without using hard drugs, while maintaining a job and stable home life, is it really helpful to judge their cannabis use? And if being high on weed all day is the best that they can manage for the rest of their lives (as some with debilitating mental, neurological, or physical conditions can reasonably claim), should we not have gratitude for the leap that they did take?

Avoiding cannabis addiction is fairly simple, and something I will get into in the following chapter.

For now, let's all agree that next time we see someone consuming what we consider to be an excessive dose of cannabis, we'll employ a little curiosity about what else is going on in their life that might warrant such behavior (while also considering what foods, social media, romance, pills, entertainment, and shopping excursions dictate our own emotional landscape). And even if we can't think of anything, we'll still mind our own fucking business.

THE (RELUCTANTLY COMPOSED) HOW-TO CHAPTER

A FEW TIPS ABOUT CANNABIS AND EXERCISE I LEARNED THE HARD WAY

FLYING BLIND

A few months after Colorado implemented its recreational cannabis program in 2014, *New York Times* op-ed writer Maureen Dowd paid Denver a visit to see what all the fuss was about. The East Coast reporter—known for her somewhat misogynistic takedowns of Hillary Clinton—was unfamiliar with marijuana culture or products and made a common rookie mistake her first night after visiting a local dispensary.

"The caramel-chocolate flavored candy bar looked so innocent, like the Sky Bars I used to love as a child," she wrote in her *New York Times* column "Don't Harsh Our Mellow, Dude." "Sitting in my hotel room in Denver, I nibbled off the end and then, when nothing happened, nibbled some more. . . . But then I felt a scary shudder go through my body and brain. I barely made it from the desk to the bed, where I lay curled up in a hallucinatory state for the next eight hours. . . . As my paranoia deepened, I became convinced that I had died and no one was telling me."

A similar scenario befell Miami Heat guard Dion Waiters in 2019. Seeking relief from a stomachache that had kept him out of a game, Waiters gobbled a blind handful of THC-infused gummies while flying to Los Angeles for a game against the Lakers. A short time later, Waiters experienced a cannabis-induced panic attack, leading someone to call the paramedics once they landed. This prevented him from playing that night and led to a ten-game suspension for violating NBA drug laws.

Even I, a seasoned cannabis aficionado, collected a handful of edible-overdose stories in my youth. During a 2003 trip to Humboldt County, California (the mecca of cannabis growing culture), I helped pluck, trim, and cure my first harvest. Afterward, we made an infused carrot cake with the leftover trimmings from the plant (which aren't as psychoactive as nugs, but, when crushed, they break down into a condensed, wildly potent powder).

I'd never consumed edibles before and naively assumed that this trim-based cake would have a weak effect. After consuming a large (unmeasured) slice, I proceeded to drink a half-dozen beers, smoke some flower, then become violently hungry and return to the cake, remembering how good it tasted. My twenty-one-year-old mind and body had no resources to process the massive volume of THC I'd consumed (which I'd guess today was at least a few hundred milligrams). We'd traveled to a DIY show on a rural farm, and once inside the barn I discovered a jam band was crucifying a Steely Dan song. Offended, I leaped onto the stage, grabbed the mic, and chastised the band for their musical insolence, before tearing my shirt off and running through a cornfield shouting, "I will lead you to the musical promised land!"

There are two things all these stories have in common: (1) None of us were paying attention to the amount of THC we were consuming; and (2) there was no experienced person looking out for us.

Prohibitionists like to point to surges in marijuana overdoses at emergency rooms following Colorado's legalization as evidence that pot is a menace. Though, as I've mentioned before, cannabis overdoses are never lethal, and the only treatment offered by a physician is hydration, monitoring, and reassurance that you're not dying. Curiously, though, when I spoke with former president of the American College of Emergency Physicians Dr. Larry Bedard when reporting on the Colorado surge in ER visits for weed, he told me that while working in hospitals in Marin County, California—where one of the highest concentrations of marijuana users in the nation lived—he "saw less than ten patients in twenty years who came in where their chief complaint was marijuana."

At a time when Colorado doctors were seeing several of these patients each day, what was it that made California's black market (this was before it was legalized) so different?

In the early days of legalization, regulations surrounding potency, labeling, and consumer education (via budtenders) was abysmal. Many edibles had inconsistent dosages, and curiosity seekers new to pot were not given proper information. When she walked into that dispensary in 2014, no one had explained to Maureen Dowd that the candy bar she'd bought contained sixteen servings, and that consuming the whole thing would be a nightmare for someone unaccustomed to it.

Waiters is reported to have been given his gummies by a teammate, and likely didn't know how much he was taking (or what kind of dose he'd need to treat his stomachache) when he'd gobbled them down.*

When we made that carrot cake in Humboldt County, we forgot to pay attention to (a) what amount of THC was in the trim we were using, (b) how much trim we were putting into the recipe, which, if we had, would've told us: (c) how medicated each slice of the cake was, and (d) what an appropriate dose would've been. We were all equally naive and, like Dowd and Waiters, were missing a key ingredient that explains the difference between California's emergency rooms and Colorado's: an experienced guide.

A fair amount of responsibility does belong to budtenders and

....

* Though I never spoke with him. Perhaps he knew what he was doing and was like, "Fuck it—let's break on through to the other side! See you in Valhalla!"

dispensaries for not providing better information on how to navigate edibles. But at the same time, we don't expect cashiers at grocery stores to break down the difference between a bottle of beer and a bottle of Everclear to their customers—despite an overdose on booze being potentially fatal.

Nearly everyone has a story of getting hammered on alcohol for the first time in their teens or twenties, vomiting like crazy, and, if you're lucky, making it to bed with only a massive hangover to worry about in the morning. In time, you (hopefully) learned from this experience—and were educated by those around you—about not drinking on an empty stomach, when to cut yourself off, and what circumstances are unsafe for drinking (e.g., anytime you have to drive yourself home).

Some people are lucky enough to grow up with parents or friends who instruct them on these basics of drinking when they're starting out. Similarly, the mass amount of stoners in California who never went to the ER were part of a community of experienced potheads who could give them tips on the appropriate dosage and when to mix it with alcohol (almost never), and to calmly explain that they'll be OK if they overdid it—thereby stopping thoughts of death and visiting the hospital in their tracks.

I understand that I'm not painting cannabis in a very favorable light here.

Despite the lack of any real physical threat, cannabis overdoses are no fun—particularly if you don't understand that you'll be fine in a few hours. But such an experience can be easily avoided with a little education and intentional consumption. The same goes for working out as well. As I mentioned in the previous chapter, excessive exercise has the potential to be just as destructive as overdoing it with other substances, so it's important to have someone with a bit of experience in both camps on your side before fusing these two together.

Ultimately, I am writing this chapter as the how-to I wish I'd had when starting out. As someone who grew up in a world of religious conmen and emotionally manipulative narcissists, I am reluctant to tell anyone how to do anything. So you're welcome to challenge or dismiss any advice given here, and I encourage you to look for other (perhaps contradictory) sources as well. It wasn't my idea to write a how-to chapter, but after giving it some thought, I certainly see the value in it.

If someone had explained to me years ago that mountain trails are often poorly marked and wildly confusing so don't get loaded up on edibles, blast Norwegian death metal on your headphones, and run ten miles into mysterious darkness with no food or water, it would've saved me a pretty rough night in the woods.

In this chapter, I will provide information for both those living in legalized states and those subsisting in a black market (as a former pot dealer from Iowa, I have some insight into these challenges), what exercises to begin with when high, where to safely work out high outdoors, how to establish what a proper dose looks like for you, what cannabis products are best for working out versus for recovery, how to navigate a dispensary, and, if necessary, how to purchase cannabis on the black market.

However, this chapter is not a guide for experienced athletes. There will be no weighing in on barefoot running, splits, or cross-training. Similarly, if you are a lifelong subscriber to *High Times* and religiously watch every episode of *Bong Appétit*, some of the following information may seem a little rudimentary.

And of course, I am legally obligated to state that I am not a doctor.

I happily encourage you to speak with your physician before trying anything in this book, and especially when it comes to this chapter.

BUYING BUD

For those of you lucky enough to live in a state that has fully legalized recreational cannabis (assuming your particular county hasn't banned it, as is the case in much of Colorado), congratulations! Take a moment of gratitude to acknowledge how lucky you are to be alive in this time and place.

If you live in one of the thirty-three states that have legalized medical cannabis, you may want to ask yourself: Do I have a health condition that can be treated with cannabis? A quick Google search can reveal the list of qualifying ailments in your state, as well as the name of a doctor who can write you a prescription.

Once you find yourself with a medical marijuana card, keep in mind that these products are infinitely cheaper (due to lower taxes) and more potent than recreational products.

If you have several dispensaries to choose from, it may be worth doing a little research on each dispensary's reputation, just like with restaurants. Yelp provides customer reviews of dispensaries, as do marijuana sites like Leafly and Weedmaps. If a particular dispensary looks good to you, google its name with the word "review," or hit the "news" tab to see if they've been busted for violating pesticide regulations, selling inconsistently dosed products, or mistreating their employees.

"I'd say about fifty percent of budtenders know what they're talking about," says Mia Jane, a cannabis educator and social media influencer.* "Some dispensaries do a really good job of educating them, but it is retail, and there's high turnover. In medical dispen-

....

* I know this term often inspires eye rolls, but influencers have become a necessary conduit of information in the industry, as cannabis companies are severely restricted in what they're allowed to say on social media. As a medical marijuana patient who got off nineteen different pharmaceutical prescriptions for chronic pain and gastric distress,

saries people come in knowing what they want, but the rec shops that cater to tourists, I'd say seventy percent of the time customers come in not knowing what they want, and they don't know what everything is or how to use it."

Mia Jane advises customers to be as transparent as possible with the budtender about your experience level and what kind of effect or treatment you're looking for. Are you using this product to enhance exercise? Recovery? Do you need it for sleep? Are you looking for a mild dose that you can still function on, or are you looking to sink deep into the couch for a lazy Sunday movie marathon?

"People should know what they're looking to get out of cannabis before they start using it," says Joanna Zeiger of the Canna Research Foundation. "Because if you don't know what you're after, how will you know if it's working?"

I personally prefer edibles over smoked flower for the body high, and while there are studies showing smoked cannabis is a bronchial dilator—opening up airways for better breathing—that doesn't necessarily mean it's the healthier choice.

"Smoking is going to introduce a whole lot of undesirable compounds, including potential carcinogens," says Dr. Ethan Russo. "It's true that people who smoke only cannabis have lower rates of lung cancer than tobacco smokers, but your body still has to metabolize that garbage. That's why I don't recommend smoking and think vaping is preferable."

For vaporization, there are devices that will vaporize your flower, and ones that come with a built-in or changeable cartridge full of cannabis oil, though most of these cartridges are made from distillates that contain only THC and no other cannabinoids.

....

Mia Jane takes her role as an educator very seriously and is often critical of companies that are not acting in the best interest of patients and customers.

"THC on its own is a lousy drug. It needs [terpenes and other cannabinoids] to round out the experience, making it much safer," adds Dr. Russo. "A lot of these extraction methods are squandering the terpenes until you end up with a pure THC product, which will get you incredibly high but is not necessarily the best approach. Those new to cannabis should try a CBD-dominant product, with low amounts of THC, which won't take you into an intergalactic state. A little bit can go a long way toward increased energy and help you get into exercise."

When it comes to edibles, Mia Jane recommends asking for a product made from cannabutter, which will retain the terpenes of the plant better than others.

"I like to use a one-to-one edible before the gym, which helps me work out longer and be less sore afterward," she says, referring to products that have an equal amount of THC and CBD. "CBD can offset the anxiety of THC, but too much can make you sleepy. I take ten milligrams of CBD throughout the day, but I'll take thirty milligrams at night and easily fall asleep."

Edibles are considerably more expensive, however. So if you're shopping on a budget, you may want to consider purchasing flower and then turn it into edibles yourself. This allows you to infuse the cannabis into a food of your choice, and teaches you a lot about the process. I personally enjoy my Ardent Nova decarboxylator for this, but there are other devices available online that can be shipped even to non-legalized states. And while this will save you money in the long term, these devices can cost a few hundred dollars. If you're unsure about this commitment, a number of blogs will instruct you on how to turn flower into edibles in your own kitchen. (Though, again, beware the pervasive smell that will follow.)

If you're on a diet, you can consider asking your budtender for an edible with healthy ingredients—which can sometimes be a challenge, as this industry insists on flooding the market with edibles made from sugary, processed foods. There are also strains and products that promise none of the appetite-inducing ("munchies") effects of most cannabis.

If you live in a state with no form of legal cannabis, well . . .

BLACK MARKET

Providing instruction on how to break the law puts myself and my publisher in some legal gray area. So, I will begin by discouraging anyone from putting themselves in legal jeopardy by purchasing black market cannabis. If the option is available to you, perhaps consider taking a trip to a legalized state—or even moving to one! (Though don't come to Denver; we're full up at the moment, thank you very much.)

However, like a high school guidance counselor handing out condoms, I accept that some people are going to break the law no matter what, and keeping them ignorant of helpful information serves no one.

If you happen to visit a legalized state, or have a friend visit one for you, returning home with these now-illicit products is still technically illegal. The Transportation Security Administration (TSA) has stated numerous times that it's not prosecuting anyone for transporting small amounts of cannabis, and unless someone tips off your local police (and they are so unburdened with legit police work they'll bust someone for returning home with a few edibles), you're not likely to get in any trouble for this.

How do I know this? Well . . . never mind.

If none of these options are available to you, it could be worth making friends with a pothead. As the *Healthy Stoner* blogger Roger

Boyd said at the beginning of this book, no matter where he was in the world, he was always able to find someone willing to sell him pot (or connect him with a source who could) simply by looking for "someone cool." (An ambiguous description, I know, but youth and counterculture clothing are a good place to start.)

I guarantee you that *someone* in your town, no matter how small or conservative, is getting high. And that person likely bought it somewhere close. If possible, try to work it into conversation that you're having trouble sleeping, or are looking for a pain-relieving alternative to aspirin, and wasn't there a story on the news last night about cannabis treating such ailments?

However, in these moments you do run the risk of sounding like a narc.

When I first moved to Denver, I spent a good ten days wandering around bars asking people, "Hey, man, you know where I can find some grass?" I sounded straight out of *21 Jump Street* and failed to procure any weed until someone mercifully explained to me, "Look, just go to Civic Center Park, and someone will try to sell you pot."

This turned out to be completely true.

However, the weed was profoundly low quality, and the experience more than a bit sketchy. I mention it here only as a last-resort effort. If you can't find anyone to connect you with a pot dealer, go to a park in the center of your nearest big city, and it'll only be a matter of time before someone approaches you with an offer. You'll likely never encounter anyone selling edibles on the black market, only raw flower. If they are selling edibles, I strongly advise against it, unless you know the person well (and even then, it's risky, due to inconsistent dosage).

If you find yourself a good, consistent dealer, it's not uncommon that they'll know a thing or two about the product they're selling you. While many will look at you blankly and say, "It's weed, it'll get you high," others will at least have a variety of sativa or indica on the menu, and maybe more. Similar to with the budtender, feel free to share with your dealer what you're using the cannabis for, and it's possible they'll have something specific to offer. In both cases, it's reasonable to ask if you can smell the cannabis. You want something with a pungent aroma, as that will tell you a lot about its potency. Also, if you're allowed to touch it (most dispensaries forbid this), you're looking for flower that is moist enough that it doesn't crumble when you gently squeeze it, but not so moist that mildew has formed (similar to old food, moldy pot will have a layer of cottony white fluff growing across it).

Like a life partner, a good dealer is hard to find. So if you get a good one, comply with whatever ground rules they set about phone communication, referrals, and how long to stay at their home. Some dealers are chatty and don't want people coming in and out quickly and drawing attention, while others would rather have a brief exchange and not bother with pleasantries.

GETTING HIGH

Now that you've safely returned home with your cannabis, it's time to develop your own getting-high ritual. If you've never consumed cannabis, or haven't in decades, I definitely recommend trying it out a few times in the safety of your own home before adding anything to the mix—particularly exercise. (And it may not be a bad idea to have a seasoned cannabis user at home with you, to avoid ending up like Maureen Dowd.)

Make sure you don't have any pressing responsibilities for the next few hours before consuming. While seasoned users can accomplish most tasks under the influence, freshmen should be advised that most activities will seem a bit strange and unwieldy when high. I recommend taking the dog for a walk and having a babysitter or partner look after the kids for a while, before ingesting anything. It might even be worth putting on some comfy clothes, setting yourself up in the living room or bedroom with some nice herbal (noncaffeinated) tea, snacks, blankets, and music or your favorite movie beforehand. Oh, and water. Plenty of water.

You can also do yourself a big favor by turning off your phone.

If you prefer smoked flower over other options, take a moment to ask yourself, Will my neighbors be able to smell this? Smoked cannabis can be profoundly pungent, and while it dissipates after several hours, if you live in an apartment building or share a house with others, you may want to open a window—and maybe even place a box fan in that window (facing outward) and blow your smoke into that. One surefire way to disguise the smell is the old college-dorm trick of stuffing a cardboard toilet paper core with dryer sheets and blowing your smoke into that. The smoke attaches to the fragrance and makes your house smell lovely.

This may all seem like overkill, but if you live in a building with a no-smoking policy, you could end up evicted over excessive pot smell (this is particularly true in public housing). Also, for anyone with children, some states will (tragically) launch a Child Protective Services investigation over cannabis use around kiddos.*

Vaporizers are a nice alternative for this reason, as they do not produce any lingering scent.

Another consideration is what device to use when smoking pot.

Rolling papers are often available anywhere tobacco products are sold, and there are plenty of tutorials online for how to roll a joint. However, it's worth noting that the end of a burning joint will waste

....

* And for anyone wondering, contact highs are very rare. Unless you're in an elevator with Willie Nelson and Snoop Dogg, it's unlikely that someone's smoke will get another person high.

some of your pot and create a lot of excess smoke. Also, pipes, bongs (i.e., "water pipes"), and chillums are increasingly available at convenience stores. Or, failing that, it's likely there's a head shop not far from you. There are blogs and tutorials for how to go about using these devices as well.

In attempting to combat the scourge of overdoses, the state of Colorado launched a PSA a few years back with the slogan "Start low and go slow." I highly recommend you heed this sage advice. When you're smoking, the cannabis takes less than a couple of minutes for the full effect to set in. So if you're new to this, I recommend you stick with one hit, wait around ten or fifteen minutes, and see how you feel. If you feel nothing, take a second hit and stick with that. It's very common for those new to cannabis to feel nothing their first few tries.

"I recommend people keep a log of what they're taking, how much, and what the effect is," says Joanna Zeiger. "Because you're not gonna remember what the effect was in three weeks when you go to the dispensary. And remember: Just because that product didn't work, doesn't mean cannabis didn't work. It's just that that product isn't right for your needs."

This same information applies to edibles with one caveat: unlike smoked flower, edibles generally take effect after around twenty to ninety minutes. This is why so many people—like Maureen Dowd—overdose on edibles and not smoked flower. They take a little, feel nothing, double the dose, and find themselves transported to a menacing realm an hour later. I recommend consuming somewhere between 1 and 5 milligrams of THC the first few times you get high, then *slooooooowly* work your way up from there.

"Edibles take longer with onset, but they also last longer," says Ethan Russo. "For a medical patient, or an endurance athlete, this is an advantage, because you don't need to medicate as much throughout the day."

Another factor is what you have in your stomach. Cannabis is either fat or alcohol soluble, and so the potency of your edibles could be impacted by some degree if you just ate a giant Thanksgiving meal or are on the end of a three-day fast. I'd recommend avoiding mixing it with alcohol, particularly if you're new to pot, as this can have a detrimental impact on your high (particularly with edibles).

Once you do feel something, no matter how mild, sit with the sensation for a moment, examining how you feel physically and emotionally. Is this a pleasurable experience? Is there an ear-to-ear grin stretched across your face? A Christmas-morning-like sensation in your belly? Does food suddenly taste extra delicious and music sound infinitely more complex and poetic?

If so, congratulations! You've reached your destination.

Do not be tempted to think that increasing your dose will increase your pleasure. This is a common problem with those new to drugs (particularly addicts in desperate search of comforting). Cannabis has a vast spectrum of effects on the human body, and recklessly increasing your dose can take you from heaven to hell if you're not careful.* As I mentioned earlier, cannabis does have a biphasic effect, meaning that a reasonable dose can provide energy, pain relief, and euphoria, but go too far and you could be in for a rough ride. This conundrum was first reported over two thousand years ago by Shen Nong Ben Cao Jing, the father of traditional Chinese medicine, who praised the myriad uses of cannabis, calling it "one of the supreme elixirs of immortality," yet said that when taken in excess, it "makes people see demons."

....

* I may be laying on the caution a bit thick here. It's not like there's a thin line between too much and too little. Like alcohol, you can be mildly over the line or extremely over the line. Typically when someone has a bad time, they took several times the recommended dose. But if you only need 10 milligrams of THC and you take 20 milligrams, you'll likely be fine, with possibly a bit of mild discomfort.

If you do feel you've taken too much—resulting in anxiety, disorientation, and increasingly dark and paranoid thoughts—remind yourself of two simple things: you're not in any danger, and you'll feel better in a few hours. Maybe write that down on a piece of paper.

And, as was mentioned at the top of this chapter, if you're the type of person prone to anxiety, you'll want to seek out a high-CBD, low-THC product beforehand.

During Neil Young's guest appearance on *The Howard Stern Show*, the shock jock confessed that he used to love getting high but had given it up after experiencing anxiety a few times. "Try black pepper balls if you get paranoid," Young told Stern. "Just chew two or three pieces. I just found this out myself. Try it."

One thing I would advise is contacting a friend long before calling 911.*

The comedian Amy Sedaris once confessed to overdoing it with some pot cookies, then attempted to call an ambulance via the intercom connected to her building's doorman. Instead of making the call, Sedaris's doorman simply talked her down through the crackly speaker, and everything was fine. This is a preferable outcome to that of the Ohio man who called 911, saying that he was "too high." When police arrived at his house, the man didn't want any medical attention; he just wanted to rat himself out as having weed in his car. Shrugging, the police accepted the man's keys, found the pot in his car, wrote him a ticket, and left.

An alternative you could consider is calling Leaf411. It's a free educational service staffed by registered nurses educated in the nuances of medical cannabis who can advise you on a variety of issues:

....

* When visiting Hunter Thompson's home years ago, I noticed a handwritten sign on the fridge exclaiming, "never call 911! this means you!" While I'm not as fundamentalist on the subject, I do think it's good advice when dealing with marijuana.

from recommending a product for your specific medical need to talking you down when you've had too much and think the sky is falling.

GETTING HIGH AND WORKING OUT

After you've been uneventfully high a few times, you can begin to incorporate other activities into the experience. If you haven't exercised in years, I wouldn't recommend leaping into your nearest CrossFit gym for some high-octane cardio. Perhaps some light stretching or beginner's yoga or aerobics might be a good primer for waking up your body from its hibernation. You can find instructional videos for either of these with a quick Google search. I enjoy Fitness Blender's free workouts, but there are a lot of options out there to choose from.

Personally, I think walking is not only the best form of exercise but the one that jives best with a cannabis high. Try a local park or somewhere in your neighborhood (if you feel safe there, particularly at night). Listening to music on headphones during a walk, with a bit of THC dancing in my veins, is my happy place.

Over the years I've found that, as with each individual's reaction to cannabis, each athlete approaches working out high a little differently. This is why Heather and Antonio DeRose of Green House Healthy recommend keeping a journal to document what strains, products, and doses, along with various workouts, fit best with your mind and body.

"This helps narrow down the proper [dose], and creates a better customized training plan," says Antonio. "It's part of our cannabis-training assessment we offer when training clients who consume cannabis before or after workouts."

"Cannabis can help some increase duration and focus while training, while also reducing pain, so being aware of how your body feels during and after the training session is something to keep a log about," adds Heather. "The first dab I did was before a HIIT class, and I found it helped me focus and reduce pain. However, this may not be the case for others, so I usually don't recommend trying a new consumption method or product before participating in a physical activity. It's really about each person finding and re-creating the desired effect for themselves, which is a process. I know some who can consume over one-hundred-milligram edibles and train for hours or run a marathon, which is not the case for myself. I would probably be stuck sitting at the starting line if I consumed edibles in that amount before a race!"

Timing your dose with your workout can also be an effective tactic to get the most out of the experience. Many of the athletes interviewed for this book, along with myself, recommend already being in an active state when your pot kicks in. This requires either taking your edible ten to twenty minutes before you begin or waiting to smoke until you're just about to or have already started your workout. In my experience, if the edible kicks in before you've even changed clothes, you're in danger of lethargy taking hold.

Similar to not trying out a new dose or product while exercising, when it comes to leaving the house, it's recommended that you stick with what's familiar. "If you're new to running high, consider running a route you've run a dozen times in the last year, so you know you won't get lost," says Avery Collins. "Otherwise, many of the new higher-end GPS watches from Suunto, Garmin, and Coros offer GPS features that will ensure you won't get lost."

As I mentioned before, my early attempts at running high on mountain trails (which also happened to be the first few times this city boy had ventured onto *any* trails) got me into a bit of trouble. It can be such an exciting, transcendent experience, and it's easy to become so lost in the hypnotic rhythms of your feet that you then literally become lost on the mountain.

Long before she became a pro ultramarathoner with an edible sponsor, Flavie Dokken once overdid it with edibles while running alone on a trail she was unfamiliar with.

"I went out in the Indian Peaks Wilderness area in the winter," she recalls. "The sun was out when I left, but the trail was snow-packed, and about three hours into my run, it started snowing and a thick fog came out. I lost track of the trail, and my only way back was to follow a creek. It took me forever with deep snow up to my knees and bushwhacking, but eventually it got me back where I started."

When running in Denver, I have intimate knowledge of every intersection, bad neighborhood, and inch of pavement in the entire metro area. But when jogging in a new city, I'm forced to turn off this autopilot and redirect some brain energy into figuring out where the fuck I am. A large factor in staying oriented in unfamiliar terrain is whether I'm listening to music or not.

TUNE IN OR TUNE OUT?

Music can be a divisive topic for many runners.

I don't think I've seen a more violently annoyed expression on someone's face than when I've been confronted by a runner or cyclist attempting to pass me on a trail who couldn't get my attention because my ears were being bathed in French house music on noise-canceling headphones. For this, Jeremy Johnson recommends keeping one ear uncovered while jogging on a trail (to hear not only other runners but also rattlesnakes), while Avery Collins recommends ditching the headphones altogether and letting the music play out loud from your phone speaker, saying, "This will allow animals to know you're coming while also allowing you to hear everything around you."

Heather and Antonio say they never listen to music while running, as they prefer to commune with their bodies and the natural setting of a trail. I hear this often from cannabis-fueled runners, and while I agree a music-free run on trails can be the meditative and safe way to go about it, it's a concession I make begrudgingly. In part this is because there is literally nothing I do in a day (writing, cooking, sex, falling asleep) that isn't accompanied by a diligently curated soundtrack. But also because I genuinely love running to music. It informs my pace and stride as much as the beats in a dance club inform how you shake your ass.

Following this hypnotic muse into the horizon can be problematic, if you're not careful.

Avery Collins often listens to psych-trance playlists while running his days-long ultraraces, but he typically waits until he's a few hours in to avoid early burnout from the overexcitement of music. "Whenever I look through the starting line and see some people with headphones on straightaway, I know who will be dropping out early," he says.

Personally, I think this can be avoided with a bit of playlist curation.

Streaming services now offer us the ability to create long, intricate playlists for a variety of needs. For me, this is the most fun part of my training regimen. Though I understand that not everyone spent their twenties writing album reviews by day while spinning records at indie dance clubs by night (like I did), and perhaps aren't tickled by the idea of organizing four-hour playlists arranged by genre, tempo, and theme. If this is the case, I invite you to pilfer any of the hundreds of workout playlists I've assembled on my Spotify account for your own weed and workout pleasure.

Part of the fun (for me, at least) is curating a playlist that matches the type of run I plan to have. Most of my playlists follow an arc of starting with one or two gentle-groove songs as my blood gets flowing, then slowly increasing in tempo over the next five or six songs, and peaking at a commanding, high-tempo sprint, before descending back down and eventually ending in a few gentle, soothing tunes (studies show listening to relaxing music post-workout aids in recovery).

But these types of playlists serve me only when I'm having a fun end-of-the-day-treat kind of run. When I'm training for a race, I'll get a little more meticulous. And, again, none of this threatens my playful attitude toward running the way competition or a training regimen can, because I honestly have so much fun doing it. Below I've included a small sampling of my favorite running-high songs, broken into three different categories.

Easy-Groove, Getting-Started Songs:
"Misty Mountain Hop," Led Zeppelin
"Unpretty," TLC
"Wig in a Box," *Hedwig and the Angry Inch* soundtrack
"A Rush and a Push and the Land Is Ours," The Smiths
"Laid," James
"Fuck You," CeeLo Green
"Hello!," *Book of Mormon* soundtrack
"Touch a Hand (Make a Friend)," Staple Singers

Mid-Tempo Medium Energy:
"Sabotage," Beastie Boys
"Rusty Cage," Johnny Cash
"Blinding Lights," The Weeknd
"Surrender," Cheap Trick

"Black Skinhead," Kanye West

"People Who Died," Jim Carroll Band

"Walking on Sunshine," Katrina and the Waves

"Movin' On Up," Primal Scream

"Nobody Speak," DJ Shadow, featuring Run the Jewels

"Inní Mér Syngur Vitleysingur," Sigur Rós

"Fight the Power," Public Enemy

"When I Grow Up," Garbage

"Green Light," Lorde

"The Chase Is Better Than the Catch," Motörhead

"Dirty Blvd," Lou Reed (live)

"Botch-a-Me," Rosemary Clooney

"Jackie," Scott Walker

"Judas," Lady Gaga

"Everything Now," Arcade Fire

Up-Tempo Sprinting:

"Town Called Malice," The Jam

"Jump into the Fire," Harry Nilsson

"Grey Seal," Elton John

"The Rat," The Walkmen

"Holland, 1945," Neutral Milk Hotel

"Rip This Joint," The Rolling Stones

"Tonight, Tonight," Smashing Pumpkins

"Master of Puppets," Metallica

"Comeback Kid," Sleigh Bells

"Dope Nose," Weezer

"The Hand That Feeds," Nine Inch Nails

"Du Hast," Rammstein

"Telstar," The Tornados

"B.O.B.," OutKast

"Poupée de Cire, Poupée de Son," France Gall
"Bat out of Hell," Meat Loaf
"Everybody's Got Something to Hide Except Me and My
   Monkey," The Beatles
"Movement," LCD Soundsystem

However, the personal connection you have with a certain song can be a deciding factor in whether it inspires you to move.

"Music taps into primitive brain structures involved with motivation, reward, and emotion," writes neuroscientist Daniel J. Levitin in *This Is Your Brain on Music*. "When we love a piece of music, it reminds us of other music we have heard, and it activates memory traces of emotional times in our lives."

Whenever I hear Ace of Base, Green Day, or any number of Christian rock bands you've likely never heard of, I'm suddenly transported back to 1997; the restless hunger of fourteen-year-old Josiah rushes through my legs, and suddenly I'm off! So you can either create your own playlist or use mine with the caveat of not judging the occasional nostalgia track.

SHOULD I TAKE MORE, OR SHOULD I COME DOWN?

This is a conundrum I often face, and I suspect most runners do as well: You're having the run of your life, and you feel better than you expected you would by this mile or hour. If you're in good shape and are familiar with your surroundings, you might find yourself wanting another tap of THC to keep this party raging.

"I like to set a distance goal, say every ten miles biking, or every two miles hiking, and reward myself with a blunt, joint, or even a dab right there in nature," says Jennessa Lea. "This may be illegal, but I fully support civil disobedience. Just ensure you are away from the trail and be respectful of families."

For most runners, a pen vaporizer or edible are more discreet and convenient options for consuming on a run. For long workouts, Avery Collins recommends dosing yourself with 5 milligrams of THC per hour (along with some CBD for inflammation or stomach cramping) and go from there. "I've tried putting THC powder in my hip water flask," says Jeremy Johnson, "but it gave me terrible cottonmouth, which is the complete opposite of what you want out of your water."

Cottonmouth during runs is one of the most common complaints I hear from those new to running high. Both Flavie Dokken and Jeremy Johnson recommend chewing gum as a remedy for this, but as someone who is strongly grossed out by gum (chiclephobia! It's a real thing! Oprah has it!), I'll just relay their recommendation and try not to think about it.

Alternatively, making sure you're well hydrated before your workout and then taking small sips of a handheld water bottle every five or ten minutes should be sufficient to avoid cottonmouth. If not, you may have medical dehydration issues worth looking into.

Working out high can be so much fun that you may be tempted to push yourself to complete collapse. This can be problematic, because it's very important to save a bit of energy for a proper cooldown and recovery. Gentle music with a bit of stretching, water, and eventually some nutritious, high-protein food (and perhaps a bit of carbs, depending on your training) are my preferred comedown accoutrements.

There are some wonderful cannabis topicals available in legalized states that can be applied to sore joints and muscles. These products typically won't get you high, as not enough THC enters the bloodstream to be effective, but will still provide anti-inflammatory relief. (Pure CBD products are an option for those without a legalized market, but they're ultimately inferior to anything with THC. A clever hack given to me by Mia Jane is to purchase the less expensive, non-psychoactive products, then mix them with your dispensary-grade THC products, as this is cheaper than buying full spectrum at the dispensary.) This is also a good time to try out some indica, CBD-heavy strains or edibles that would otherwise leave you too sedated for ambitious activity.

"I love having one rolled up and ready for me after a workout," says Jennessa. "For me, it's a fantastic reward system and helps me to push harder just knowing it's there, waiting to help melt away my pain and help aid in recovery."

AVOIDING TOLERANCE (AND ADDICTION)

When Paul McCartney recorded "Got to Get You into My Life" in 1966, few at the time knew this love song was about weed. Though after being busted several times around the world (spending a week in a Tokyo jail for his half pound of "personal use" grass), it became obvious that McCartney wasn't kidding when he said he wanted to get high "every single day of my life."

When I first discovered cannabis could act as an escape hatch from the constant anxiety, insecurity, and general dullness of life in cold, conservative Iowa, I had the same impulse as McCartney (who was about the same age as me in the mid-sixties): *Why not see the world through weed-tinted glasses all day, every day?* Though turning your cannabinoid receptors into your overworked, on-demand servants, expected to fully turn your mood around at any given moment of the day, will almost certainly lead to a spiral of dependence, preventing you from ever achieving any genuine "high."

Now, I realize this does contradict what I said in the previous chapter about not judging anyone's consumption habits. Though that was in reference to those with debilitating physical or psychological conditions that warrant daily cannabis use, who without it would be using alcohol, opioids, or some other pharmaceutical with far nastier side effects than pot.

Everyone's endocannabinoid system is impacted by various genetic, environmental, lifestyle, and psychological factors, creating a wildly complex set of variables that make up your personal cannabis tolerance. Requiring a supremely large or small volume of cannabis is nothing to be ashamed of. (In fact, if you need only a small amount, you'll save yourself quite a bit of money.) Though if you naturally require only a small dose but gradually chase some elusive sensation that you think a larger dose will provide, only to find yourself spending half your paycheck at the dispensary, you will never find what you're after. Trust me.

For those who simply enjoy cannabis recreationally, or are using it to enhance their workout, I highly recommend avoiding daily use. I'm not saying never wake-and-bake (the cannabis equivalent of brunch mimosas) or never be stoned all day every now and again. I'm just recommending that you pay attention to the volume and frequency of your consumption so as to avoid acquiring any kind of tolerance.

"Make it a treat," comedian Sarah Silverman says of her cannabis use. "Just because you like something doesn't mean it needs to become your whole thing. Because then it's not fun anymore."

Also, a study out of CU Boulder revealed that after a certain point of cannabis consumption, the euphoric impact of THC reaches its peak, regardless of how much additional cannabis is consumed. Yet the negative impacts (anxiety, lethargy, short-term memory impairment) will continue to climb. As someone who was once twenty-two, I understand the thrill of finding out just how much weed you can smoke (I consumed a whole quarter ounce in one sitting at that age, just to see what would happen), but let me tell you from experience, this is not a smart move. (Again, if you have a serious medical condition, your daily dosage is between you and your doctor. I am not a doctor. I'm just an aging stoner with some wisdom to pass along.)

If you do find yourself wondering when the last time was that you *weren't high*, I highly recommend taking a break. I understand if this causes your anti-authority, fuck-you-I-won't-do-what-you-tell-me hackles to rise up. And that's fine. I get the same way when anyone tells me I can't be a productive writer, or runner, as a pothead. But this is just my recommendation. Also, this doesn't require any big declaration to the world of your newfound sobriety. In fact, I'd recommend not telling anyone you're taking a break. Just do it for yourself and set your own parameters. Whether that means delaying your next high for a few hours, days, or weeks is up to you.

I've intentionally written this book—and this chapter especially—without ever explicitly telling you, dear reader, to always do this and never do that. I'm merely reporting on the tactics that have worked for myself and other cannabis athletes, along with a little scientific context. Ultimately, you are in the driver's seat of this vehicle, and the responsibility is yours alone to learn what safe and healthy looks like for you.

Like Charles Barkley, I am not a role model.

I'm just a guy who likes to get stoned and run.

PROMISES TO KEEP, AND MILES TO GO BEFORE WE SLEEP

Running's always been a big thing in our family. Especially running away from the police.

—*The Loneliness of the Long Distance Runner*

IT'S ELECTION NIGHT IN AMERICA...

While tallying the presidential results is likely to be a long, boring slog—randomly punctuated by an anxious drip of esoteric details—there is one landslide being called early in the evening: weed. Voters in five states passed cannabis-reform ballot measures tonight; a resounding, bipartisan indictment of the war on drugs not seen since 2016, when eight states gave this industry the green light.

New Jersey is one of the more exciting states legalizing recreational marijuana. When it launches its industry next year, it will inadvertently force the hand of New York City to implement full legalization, along with others along the eastern seaboard.* Voters in traditionally Republican-dominated states like Arizona, South Dakota, Montana, and *Mississippi, for Christ's sake,* also gave an enthusiastic thumbs-up to pot tonight.

I just drove twelve hours from Denver to my hometown in Iowa, listening as the results trickled in over the radio. My dad is having knee-replacement surgery, and I've come home to bring him a buffet of CBD-rich anti-inflammatory creams, edibles, tinctures, and smokable flower for his recovery. As I watch the promising news on his TV, I'm hoping my dad will live long enough to buy all of this at his local dispensary, so I don't have to haul it across three states.

....

* Washington, DC, actually legalized rec in 2014, but because Congress controls the DC budget, no funding was ever approved for a cannabis regulatory agency, which would be needed to establish a legal cannabis market. Weed politics is really weird.

It feels inevitable now.

Not wanting to feel left out, the governor of Virginia the following week will announce his intention to lead the way to legalizing recreational cannabis in his state, followed by Israel's justice minister, saying the nation will roll out its rec program in a mere nine months.

Approval for full legalization is now at 68 percent (medical is even higher), which is double what it was twenty years earlier when I flunked out of high school. I am not surprised the falling dominoes are gaining speed. What has shocked me is the role that cannabis has played throughout the COVID-19 crisis.

Throughout this pandemic, the rallying cry of Republicans has been "Democrats want to keep marijuana stores open and churches closed." And they weren't wrong!

When Colorado went into lockdown in March, people began stocking up on weed like it was toilet paper, creating a health hazard in the form of desperately long lines. This led our governor, Jared Polis (a former congressman, arguably one of the biggest advocates for cannabis reform in congressional history), to immediately declare dispensaries an "essential business," right alongside pharmacies and grocery stores.

Other governors of legalized states instantly followed suit.

I was standing on the sidewalk in one of these gargantuan lines outside a dispensary when this news flashed across my phone. When I finished reading, I looked up and saw the intersection of Colfax and Broadway, where I used to buy shitty weed from a stranger who wouldn't make eye contact. It was one of those moments when it felt good to be growing old and seeing history unfurl.

Around the same time, former NFL player Kyle Turley received a cease-and-desist letter from the FDA for claiming his CBD product, Neuro XPF, could boost users' immune systems and help fight COVID-19. Even cannabis-reform advocates criticized him for this, as the movement is often discredited by claims of a panacea. A short time later, though, a variety of studies began to show that CBD, THC, and various terpenes could, in fact, be used to treat COVID-19 in a variety of ways—and could even prevent its most deadly complications.

A few weeks after this, Nancy Pelosi was taking flak from Republicans for inserting a cannabis banking provision* into a COVID-19 relief bill. "I don't agree that cannabis is not related to this," she said when asked about it in a press conference. "[Cannabis] is a therapy that has proven successful."

In such a short time, purchasing cannabis went from a sketchy crime to an essential business, its medical prowess from a fringe theory to being argued for by the Speaker of the House during a national crisis.

We've certainly come a long way from the days of Anslinger, Nixon, and Reagan. The ideas of *Reefer Madness* are nothing more than a punch line today (even among cannabis detractors), and the cannapocalypse promised by fearmongering conservatives leading up to legalization never came to fruition.

Economic fears that legalization would ruin our reputation and our desirability have not only failed to materialize but have proved just the opposite. Colorado tourism is booming louder than ever (or at least it was pre-COVID-19), numerous studies show that when a city legalizes cannabis, home values tend to skyrocket, and Denver's population has only soared in the last eight years.

The only thing not soaring is cannabis use among youth.

Even President Trump's own anti-drug National Marijuana

---

* Due to the federal illegality of cannabis, banks are reluctant to have any dealings with the cannabis industry, preventing a lot of businesses from obtaining loans or even getting business accounts, resulting in a massive amount of cash moving through this $40 billion industry.

Initiative office admitted that since Colorado implemented legalization in 2014, cannabis use among twelve-to-seventeen-year-olds fell from 12.5 to 9 percent (before that it had been on the rise), and that is consistent with other legalized states. Meanwhile, twenty-one-year-old college students are, statistically, far less likely to engage in binge drinking in states with legal cannabis—a change that offers communities a decrease in violence and an increase in health and productivity.

After stoned kids, the hysteria surrounding stoned drivers was probably the most common objection to legalization. "What's to keep someone from getting all potted-up on weed and getting behind the wheel?" *Fox & Friends'* Steve Doocy bemoaned at the time.

Well, an exhaustive study published in the *Journal of Traffic Injury Prevention* showed that vehicle fatalities have actually *decreased* in states following legalization of cannabis. "Overall, these findings do not suggest an elevated risk of motor vehicle crashes associated with cannabis legalization," the study's authors wrote.

All of this is obvious to the residents of Colorado, 71 percent of whom see legalization as either a complete success or more of a success than a failure.

A survey of 827 respondents from Eaze and *Playboy* magazine found that, during the quarantine, 75 percent of respondents admitted to integrating cannabis into their sex lives—more often with edibles than smoke—with many experiencing an increase in satisfaction. Further surveys are revealing cannabis to be increasingly popular among those suffering from multiple sclerosis, obsessive-compulsive disorder, and menopause.

As cannabis becomes more accepted by every living demographic of humanity, and as science validates what history reveals as a profoundly long list of ailments that cannabis treats (and activities it enhances), *and* as legalization spreads around the world and humanity is finally reunited with this miracle plant that has been with us for twelve thousand years, one can easily assume that all the insidious harm of the war on drugs has been undone, right?

Wrong.

In nearly every legalization campaign over the last decade, the racist and classist legacies of the war on drugs have been selling points for dismantling these laws. But once the bills are signed and the investment floodgates open, the conviction for social justice tends to fizzle into the ether.

It was only in 2020 that, FBI data shows, cannabis arrests began to go down for the first time in years; yet the racial dynamics of these arrests have not changed. (Additionally, there were still more cannabis arrests in 2019 than arrests for violent crimes in the previous *four years put together.*) According to the ACLU, Black Americans are still arrested at four times the rate of white Americans for marijuana infractions—despite these groups using cannabis at equal rates. Even in a place like DC, which "legalized" in 2014, Black people account for 90 percent of the arrests for issues like public consumption, despite only making up 45 percent of the population.

Currently, one in five in the US prison population is incarcerated for a marijuana offense, according to the National Center for Drug Abuse Statistics, most of them for doing the same thing that is currently making the rich a lot richer in places like Colorado.

Back in 2009, Kayvan Khalatbari could launch Denver Relief with four grand and a half pound of weed. Today, due to extraordinary taxes, fees, and regulations, it costs at least $800,000 just to get a cannabis business off the ground (with no expectation to turn a profit for a few years). Because of federal prohibition, cannabis businesses aren't allowed to file for the galaxy of tax deductions most businesses take for granted. And banks aren't willing to risk federal prosecution by loaning money to any cannabis business. So the market is accessible only to those with a few mil already in the bank, and the ability to wait a few years before collecting a paycheck. And guess what they look like?

Currently, Black people make up only 4 percent of the cannabis market ownership, while it's over 80 percent for their Caucasian counterparts—many of whom don't even like cannabis.

While attending a cannabis investor conference in Denver, I met loads of money-minded old white dudes who openly admitted they thought pot was a dangerous drug that should never have been legalized but nevertheless saw an investment opportunity. Beyond my disagreeing with their assessment of cannabis, I kept thinking, *You're willing to bankroll a substance you believe is harmful to society in order to make money for yourself? Isn't that, like, the definition of evil?*

At the same time, the professional underground growers—many of whom take pride in the medical nuance of their product, have been caring for the sick for generations, and have contributed a great deal to the legalization movement—often can't enter the legal market because of prohibitions against anyone with a criminal record receiving a license to open a business, or even work a low-level job like trimming. Meanwhile, the well-financed philistines dominating this $40 billion industry (projected to reach anywhere from $70 to $130 billion by 2024.) care nothing for the medical value of their products, focusing only on high-THC products that'll "fuck you up!" but contain little to no terpenes or other cannabinoids.

"The rules of the industry are made by politicians, not scientists," says Dr. Ethan Russo. "And don't look to politics to make an informed decision about what's best for the consumer."

Now that big-name Republicans like former Speaker of the House John Boehner are getting into the industry, it's unsettling that some of the profits are going to people who support (vocally, if not financially) the law enforcement and prison-industrial complex that continues to persecute underground growers (who actually care about the product) and people of color—particularly when those same people of color make up half the consumers of the product.

"If we're not careful, we could lose this industry to only the big players, who will treat it like Big Pharma, stripping all the cannabinoids into separate products," adds Mia Jane. "And that can strip the plant of many of its benefits, because these cannabinoids need to interact with each other for an entourage effect. And that's why education is important, and creating a community that cares about this plant and is involved in how the industry treats it."

I don't want to suggest there isn't a valiant effort to change all this.

Earlier this year former NBA star Al Harrington launched his business-incubator program for one hundred Black cannabis entrepreneurs. "I feel like the war on drugs was aimed towards our community, and they used cannabis as pretty much the main drug to continue to lock us up," Harrington told CNBC when launching the program. "All this money being made now, we're not represented; we're not there. And I feel like we pioneered this industry."

Organizations like the Minority Cannabis Business Association and the Cannabis Cultural Association have been bringing a lot of attention to this issue, speaking with policy makers and empowering disenfranchised communities with the tools they need to break into the industry. While running for the Democratic presidential nomination, Bernie Sanders pledged in 2019 to federally legalize cannabis in his first one hundred days, expunge all marijuana convictions, and provide $20 billion in grants to "entrepreneurs of color who continue to face discrimination in access to capital" and $10 billion in grants for businesses "that are at least 51 percent owned or controlled by those in disproportionately impacted areas or individuals who have been arrested for or convicted of marijuana offenses."

Though, for a variety of reasons, this was not enough to win him the nomination.

Instead, we settled for Joe Biden, often credited as an architect of the war on drugs, 1990s edition, as well as the only Democratic candidate to not run on full legalization, while randomly tossing out the "gateway drug" theory and "we need more research" rhetoric on the campaign trail when asked about cannabis. Yet his promise to decriminalize pot on the federal level and expunge marijuana convictions was still the most progressive cannabis platform of any major party candidate in US history—showing you just how much pressure there is on Washington to address this issue.

I know this comes as a wet blanket after all that talk about how fun weed is, particularly with running. But this is important shit. I don't know about you, but I have a difficult time enjoying myself if I know my pleasure is coming at the expense of someone else's pain. When running the Colfax Marathon back in 2015, I was having the time of my life running high through a city that held so much love and memories for me . . . until the course took us past the Denver County Jail.

Even though we'd legalized, and incarcerations for marijuana had been plummeting for years, there were surely a decent number of people locked up in there for some marijuana infraction (or perhaps a different charge that still had connections to the war on drugs)—and they likely didn't look like me, or anyone surrounding me in the race. After that, it became difficult to stay present and soak up the positive energy radiating around me.

Sure, the sun was shining, my anandamide was flowing, I'd had a good night's sleep; and my breakfast of gourmet coffee, omelet, sweet potatoes, and a 20-milligram edible was fueling my legs into a harmonious cycle of energy and momentum; and yet . . . I couldn't help but wonder what the conditions in that jail were like. How did they sleep last night? What did they have for breakfast? How much joy could they expect in their day?

And if taking an eagle's-eye view of their lives and mine, how much of my joy and how much of their misery was a reflection of our own personal behavior, and how much was simply an echo of racist drug policies launched decades before any of us were even born?

To be clear, feeling like shit about this won't help anyone. Being grateful for finding yourself running high in the sunshine instead of being clubbed in a cell doesn't make you a bad person. But, like Avery Collins said to me about play versus ambition, "It's all about keeping a balance." Let's celebrate the gains we've made as a society (educating ourselves on racism in the war on drugs, accepting the vast medical applications for cannabis, and legalizing it) while acknowledging how far we still have to go (turning awareness into action on racist laws and enforcement, creating opportunities for low-income and POC ganjapreneurs, and eliminating the "lazy stoner" trope from our culture).

I don't have all the answers, and neither do you.

For now, let's just keep our red eyes open and keep running forward.

See you on the trails.

ACKNOWLEDGMENTS

BACK WHEN THE SUBJECT OF running high (and my love of it) was only a goofy conversation stimulator at parties, there were three journalists who repeatedly insisted that it would make a great book: Scott Carney, Joel Warner, and Jayme Moye, without your encouragement, I may never have gotten this project off the ground. My enchanting partner, Anna Vandegrift, was a constant source of comfort and wisdom throughout this process, as was my editor, Michelle Howry, whose joy and enthusiasm saw me through a lot of self-doubt. It must be noted that my agent, Laura Nolan, took on this project (and the backwoods dandy who came with it) when most of the industry refused to take it (or me) seriously. Mason Tvert was a reliable political nerd whenever one was needed, as was Meghan Hicks when it came to the world of trail running. Thanks to Matt LeBarge and Allison Housley for lending me their cozy mountain cabin, where portions of this book were written, and similarly to Anita Thompson for hosting me at Hunter's legendary Owl Farm. Mia Jane connected me with so many of the key characters in this book, I shudder to imagine what it would look like without her. I've read Shea Gunther's MJToday Media newsfeed every morning for four years now, and couldn't have assembled the catalog of cannabis athletics news stories that make up much of this book without it.

ACKNOWLEDGMENTS

Special thanks to Ethan Russo, Johannes Fuss, and Greg Gerdeman for guiding me through the jungle of cannabis science (double thanks to Ethan for encouraging me to limit the m-word in this book). Martin Lee's book *Smoke Signals* was a rich source of cannabis history. Alex Hutchison's *Endure*, Bernd Heinrich's *Why We Run*, and, naturally, Christopher McDougall's *Born to Run* shaped my perception of running as much as the act itself. Big thanks to the Queen City Cooperative for opening your home and hearts to me and listening to my cannabis athletics rants every Monday night at dinner. Thesaurus.com, I'd be nothing without you. And finally, I must send love to Suspect Press, the arts and literature company I abandoned to write this book. I miss you every day.

NOTES

. . . .

INTRODUCTION: A SNOB WAITS IN LINE

5 **68 percent approving of its legalization:** Megan Brenan, "Support for Legal Marijuana Inches Up to New High of 68%," Gallup, November 9, 2020, https://news.gallup.com/poll/323582/support-legal-marijuana -inches-new-high.aspx.

9 **95 percent of Americans can't be bothered:** US Department of Health and Human Services, "Healthy People 2030," http://www.healthypeople .gov/2020/default.aspx.

CHAPTER 1: POT MAKES EXERCISE FUN

28 **"about eighty-five percent of the NBA":** "The World's Best Athletes Smoke Weed. These Are Their Stories," *Bleacher Report*, April 4, 2018, http://420.bleacherreport.com/.

28 **defensive end Chris Long:** Dave Zangaro, "Chris Long Admits to Marijuana Use, Speaks Out Against NFL Policy," NBC Sports, May 22, 2019, https://www.nbcsports.com/philadelphia/eagles/chris-long-admits -marijuana-use-speaks-out-against-nfls-policy-and-hes-right.

28 **wide receiver Calvin Johnson:** Dan Reilly, "Retired NFL Players Calvin Johnson and Rob Sims Want to Treat CTE and Pain with Marijuana—and Help from Harvard," *Fortune*, January 19, 2020, https://fortune.com /2020/01/19/calvin-johnson-rob-sims-detroit-lions-marijuana-harvard -primitive/.

28 **triggered by massive crowds:** Ritchie Whitt, "Cowboys Ex David Irving 1-on-1: 'Marijuana Can Make This World a Better Place,'" *Sports Illustrated*, February 11, 2020, https://www.si.com/nfl/cowboys/news/cowboys-ex -david-irving-1-on-1-marijuana-can-make-this-world-a-better-place.

28 **smokes a blunt before announcing his retirement:** Clarence E. Hill Jr., "How Many Games Has Cowboys DE David Irving Played 'High' In? All

of Them, He Writes," *Fort Worth Star-Telegram*, August 18, 2018, https://www.star-telegram.com/sports/nfl/dallas-cowboys/article216967150.html.

29 **while they played sober:** Patrick Anderson, *High in America* (New York: Viking, 1981), 30.

29 **list of prohibited substances:** Jeff Passan, "MLB: Players Still Subject to Penalty for Using Pot," ESPN, February 28, 2020, https://www.espn.com/mlb/story/_/id/28804440/mlb-players-subject-penalty-using-pot.

29 **several players for cannabis use:** Rex Hoggard, "PGA Tour Should Consider Marijuana for Its Use, Not as 'Drug of Abuse,'" Golf Channel, October 31, 2019, https://www.golfchannel.com/news/pga-tour-should-consider-marijuana-its-use-not-drug-abuse.

29 **releasing a statement denouncing CBD:** Kyle Jaeger, "PGA Issues Warning to Golfers Using CBD Products," *Marijuana Moment*, April 2, 2019, https://www.marijuanamoment.net/pga-issues-warning-to-golfers-using-cbd-products/.

29 **WWE wrestler Enzo Amore:** Louis Dangoor, "Enzo Amore Says Half the WWE Locker Room Smokes Marijuana," *Wrestle Talk*, January 23, 2020, https://wrestletalk.com/news/enzo-amore-says-half-the-wwe-locker-room-smokes-marijuana/.

31 **alongside accusations of sexual assault:** Jeremy Longman, "A Running Club Is 100 Miles Outside the Mainstream," *New York Times*, July 28, 1997, https://www.nytimes.com/1997/07/28/sports/a-running-club-is-100-miles-outside-of-the-mainstream.html.

33 **less likely to get cancer:** Thomas Clark, "Scoping Review and Meta-Analysis Suggests that Cannabis Use May Reduce Cancer Risk in the United States," *Cannabis and Cannabinoid Research*, August 21, 2020, https://doi.org/10.1089/can.2019.0095.

33 **lower mortality rates when experiencing heart failure:** Temitope Ajibawo, "Congestive Heart Failure Hospitalizations and Cannabis Use Disorder (2010–2014): National Trends and Outcomes," *Cureus*, July 2, 2020, https://pubmed.ncbi.nlm.nih.gov/32766001/.

33 **than those who didn't:** Sharon Sznitman, "Medical Cannabis and Cognitive Performance in Middle to Old Adults Treated for Chronic Pain," National Library of Medicine, September 2020, https://pubmed.ncbi.nlm.nih.gov/32964502/.

CHAPTER 2: CAN CANNABIS AND COMPETITION COEXIST?

42 **"most abrupt of all the mountain ranges":** "San Juan Mountains," *Colorado Encyclopedia*, https://coloradoencyclopedia.org/article/san-juan-mountains.

48 **great deal of private land:** "Rights of Way and Accessing Land," Gov.uk, https://www.gov.uk/right-of-way-open-access-land/use-public-rights -of-way.

CHAPTER 3: THE HAPPY CHEMICAL

71 **dating back to 2700 BC:** Ethan B. Russo, "Phytochemical and Genetic Analyses of Ancient Cannabis from Central Asia," *Journal of Experimental Botany*, January 2008, https://www.ncbi.nlm.nih.gov/pmc/articles /PMC2639026/.

71 **as did the Greeks:** Ethan B. Russo, "History of Cannabis and Its Preparations in Saga, Science, and Sobriquet," Wiley Online Library, August 2007, https://onlinelibrary.wiley.com/doi/abs/10.1002/cbdv .200790144.

72 **used it to lower anxiety:** Martin A. Lee, *Smoke Signals: A Social History of Marijuana—Medical, Recreational, and Scientific* (New York: Simon & Schuster, 2012), 5.

72 **plant medicines in 700 BC:** Julie Holland, *The Pot Book: A Complete Guide to Cannabis, Inner Traditions* (Rochester, VT: Bear, 2010), http:// www.drholland.com/pdfs/pot-book/bennett.pdf.

72 **Jewish rituals in ancient Israel:** "'Cannabis Burned During Worship' by Ancient Israelites—Study," BBC, May 29, 2020, https://www.bbc.com /news/world-middle-east-52847175.

72 **written on hemp paper:** Lee, *Smoke Signals*, 18.

72 **Mary Todd ate hash:** Ibid., 33.

74 **fifteenth-century Persians:** Evan Rosenberg, "Cannabinoids and Epilepsy," National Library of Medicine, August 2015, https://www.ncbi .nlm.nih.gov/pmc/articles/PMC4604191/.

76 **"from the god Shiva":** Lee, *Smoke Signals*, 4.

76 **regulates our systems of sleep:** Lu Hui-Chen and Ken Mackie, "An Introduction to the Endogenous Cannabinoid System," National Library of Medicine, April 2016, https://www.ncbi.nlm.nih.gov/pmc/articles /PMC4789136/.

77 **"essentially all human diseases":** Pál Pacher, "Modulating the Endocannabinoid System in Human Health and Disease: Successes and Failures," National Library of Medicine, May 2013, https://www.ncbi.nlm .nih.gov/pmc/articles/PMC3684164/.

92 **prodigiously throughout the day:** Dominik Wujastyk, "Cannabis in Traditional Indian Herbal Medicine," https://www.academia.edu /188844/Cannabis_in_Traditional_Indian_Herbal_Medicine_pre _publication_draft.

92 **improved night vision:** Ethan B. Russo et al., "Cannabis Improves Night Vision: A Case Study of Dark Adaptometry and Scotopic Sensitivity in Kif Smokers of the Rif Mountains of Northern Morocco," National Library of Medicine, July 2004, https://pubmed.ncbi.nlm.nih.gov/15182912/.

92 **mundane, tedious labor:** Sidney Cohen, "Working Men and Ganja: Marihuana Use in Rural Jamaica," *JAMA*, 1982, https://jamanetwork .com/journals/jama/article-abstract/379686.

92 **Zulu warriors would consume cannabis:** Lee, *Smoke Signals,* 14.

92 **rats exposed to moderate doses:** Adriaan W. Bruijnzeel, "Behavioral Characterization of the Effects of Cannabis Smoke and Anandamide in Rats," National Library of Medicine, April 2016, https://www.ncbi.nlm.nih .gov/pmc/articles/PMC4827836/.

93 **only 5 percent of the US population:** US Department of Health and Human Services, "Facts and Statistics: Physical Activity," https://www.hhs .gov/fitness/resource-center/facts-and-statistics/index.html.

CHAPTER 4: LET'S FORGET PHYSICAL

107 **anandamide is an essential component of our memory:** Eliot D. Mock, "Discovery of a NAPE-PLD Inhibitor that Modulates Emotional Behavior in Mice," *Nature Chemical Biology*, May 11, 2020, https://www.nature .com/articles/s41589-020-0528-7.

107 **other failing neurotransmitters:** Jacob D. Meyer, "Serum Endocannabinoid and Mood Changes After Exercise in Major Depressive Disorder," National Library of Medicine, September 2019, https:// pubmed.ncbi.nlm.nih.gov/30973483/.

107 **treatment for veterans suffering:** Mallory J. E. Loflin, "A Cross-Sectional Examination of Choice and Behavior of Veterans with Access to Free Medicinal Cannabis," National Library of Medicine, May 2019, https://pubmed.ncbi.nlm.nih.gov/31135227/.

128 **inflammation but muscle spasticity:** Anna Maria Malfitano, "Cannabinoids in the Management of Spasticity Associated with Multiple Sclerosis," National Library of Medicine, October 2008, https://www .ncbi.nlm.nih.gov/pmc/articles/PMC2626929/.

CHAPTER 5: IS CANNABIS A PERFORMANCE-ENHANCING DRUG?

136 **30 percent of those who take them:** National Institute on Drug Abuse, "Opioid Overdose Crisis," https://www.drugabuse.gov/drug-topics /opioids/opioid-overdose-crisis.

137 **"safest drugs known to medicine":** Martin A. Lee, *Smoke Signals: A Social History of Marijuana—Medical, Recreational, and Scientific* (New York: Simon & Schuster, 2012), 342.

148 **13 percent of US medical schools:** David Bearman, "Most Medical Schools Don't Cover the Endocannabinoid System, They All Should," *Huffington Post*, October 28, 2017, https://www.huffpost.com/entry/most -medical-schools-dont-cover-the-endocannabinoid_b_5a1de2bae 4b0e9a1b9c7b49e.

159 **Black Major League Baseball:** Richard E. Lapchick, *The 2020 Racial and Gender Report Card*, Institute for Diversity and Ethics in Sport, August 28, 2020, 9, https://43530132-36e9-4f52-811a-182c7a91933b.filesusr.com /ugd/138a69_bf76658308a34d249b61e044f575a6fd.pdf.

159 **Brewers pitcher Jeremy Jeffress:** Mike Jones, "The Sad Saga of Jeremy Jeffress," *Bleacher Report*, July 8, 2009, https://bleacherreport.com /articles/214149-the-sad-saga-of-jeremy-jeffress.

160 **which are 74 percent Black:** Christina Gough, "Share of NBA Players 2010–2020, by Ethnicity," Statista, August 28, 2020, https://www .statista.com/statistics/1167867/nba-players-ethnicity/.

160 **and 70 percent Black, respectively:** Robert W. Turner II, *Not for Long: The Life and Career of the NFL Athlete* (New York: Oxford University Press, 2018), 121.

160 **Ricky Williams was derailed:** Emily Kaplan, "How Weed Became 'Whatever': Leagues Are Ditching Old Policies," ESPN, April 30, 2020, https://www.espn.com/nfl/story/_/id/29114415/future-marijuana-drug -policy-nfl-pro-sports.

160 **Cowboys defensive end Randy Gregory:** David Moore, "'This Is Not a Character Issue'—the Story Behind Randy Gregory's Marijuana Use, Personality," *Dallas News*, February 26, 2019, https://www.dallasnews .com/sports/cowboys/2019/02/27/flashback-this-is-not-a-character-issue -the-story-behind-randy-gregory-s-marijuana-use-personality/.

160 **Laremy Tunsil is believed:** Lindsay H. Jones, "Laremy Tunsil Slides After Bong Video Surfaces, OL Says He Took Money from Ole Miss Coach," *USA Today*, April 28, 2016, https://www.usatoday.com/story /sports/nfl/draft/2016/04/28/laremy-tunsil-video-marijuana-twitter-nfl -draft/83678590/.

160 **The NBA is arguably even worse:** Kaplan, "How Weed Became 'Whatever.'"

160 **NBA All-Star Cliff Robinson:** "Cliff Robinson Demands an Apology from Portland Mayor," NBC Sports, June 8, 2020, https://www.nbcsports .com/northwest/portland-trail-blazers/cliff-robinson-demands-apology -portland-mayor-ted-wheeler-racial-profiling.

161 **Super Bowl champion Bashaud Breeland:** Tina Burnside and Leah Asmelash, "Bashaud Breeland, Kansas City Chiefs Cornerback, Arrested for Possession of Marijuana and Resisting Arrest," CNN, April 29, 2020,

https://www.cnn.com/2020/04/29/us/breeland-kansas-city-chiefs-arrest
-trnd/index.html.

161 **solidarity with Black Lives Matter:** Rick Bonnell, "NBA Players Wield
Their Power with Boycott in Ways 'Black Lives Matters' Shirts Couldn't,"
Charlotte Observer, August 27, 2020, https://www.charlotteobserver.com
/sports/charlotte-hornets/article245275495.html.

161 **two weeks out of the year:** Ken Belson, "N.F.L. Bows to Marijuana's
New Status," *New York Times*, April 16, 2020, https://www.nytimes.com
/2020/04/13/sports/football/nfl-marijuana-policy.html.

161 **be tested for cannabis:** Dan Feldman, "Report: NBA Won't Test Players
for Marijuana in Disney World Bubble," NBC Sports, June 9, 2020, https://
nba.nbcsports.com/2020/06/09/report-nba-wont-test-players-for
-marijuana-in-disney-world-bubble/.

162 **NCAA will also increase:** Brendan Bures, "Universities Worry College
Athletes Might Partner with Marijuana Brands," Fresh Toast, July 12,
2019, https://thefreshtoast.com/cannabis/universities-worry-college
-athletes-might-partner-with-marijuana-brands/.

162 **CBS killed a medical marijuana ad:** Chavie Lieber, "This Rejected
Super Bowl Ad Highlights America's Complicated Relationship with
Marijuana," *Vox*, February 3, 2019, https://www.vox.com/the-goods/2019
/1/28/18200875/acreage-medical-marijuana-super-bowl-53-ad.

CHAPTER 6: THIS IS YOUR BRAIN ON DRUGS

178 **"60 percent of the addicts":** Johann Hari, "The Hunting of Billie
Holiday," *Politico*, January 17, 2015, https://www.politico.com/magazine
/story/2015/01/drug-war-the-hunting-of-billie-holiday-114298.

179 **Anslinger himself publicly declared:** Harry Anslinger, "Organized
Protection Against Organized Predatory Crime—Peddling of Narcotic
Drugs, IV," *Journal of Criminal Law and Criminology* 636 (1933), https://
scholarlycommons.law.northwestern.edu/jclc/vol24/iss3/9/.

179 **"Mexicans, Greeks, Turks, Filipinos":** Martin A. Lee, *Smoke Signals: A
Social History of Marijuana—Medical, Recreational, and Scientific* (New
York: Simon & Schuster, 2012), 51.

179 **"its cruel and devastating forms":** Doug Sneed, *Reefer Madness:
Revisited* (self-pub., 2008), 3.

179 **"as good as white men":** Harry Anslinger, *The Protectors: The
Heroic Story of the Narcotics Agents, Citizens, and Officials in Their
Unending, Unsung Battles Against Organized Crime in America and
Abroad* (New York: Farrar, Straus and Giroux, 2017), 183; Sneed, *Reefer
Madness: Revisited*, 183.

179 **"sexual relations with negroes!":** Lee, *Smoke Signals*, 52.

180 **nefarious communist plot to incapacitate Americans:** Ibid., 62.

180 **John Ehrlichman, advisor to President Nixon:** Tom LoBianco, "Report: Aide Says Nixon's War on Drugs Targeted Blacks, Hippies," CNN, March 24, 2016, https://www.cnn.com/2016/03/23/politics/john-ehrlichman -richard-nixon-drug-war-blacks-hippie/index.html.

182 **"the mongrelization of the white race":** Curt Johnson, *500 Years of Obscene—and Counting* (St. Louis: December Press, 1997), 1.

182 **"one-sided nature of our hearings":** Lee, *Smoke Signals,* 62.

182 **When the monkeys wound up with brain damage:** Ibid., 138.

183 **addicted to injected morphine:** John H. Halpern and David Blistein, "America's War on Drugs Has Treated People Unequally Since Its Beginning," *Time,* August 12, 2019, https://time.com/5638316/war-on -drugs-opium-history/.

183 **Nixon was often so sloshed:** Leonard Garment, "Life Inside a White House that Leaks Like the Titanic," *Los Angeles Times,* March 8, 1998, https://www.latimes.com/archives/la-xpm-1998-mar-08-op-26717-story .html.

184 **scrubbed from NIDA databases:** Lee, *Smoke Signals,* 162.

186 **she was heavily addicted:** Donnie Radcliffe, "Patti Davis Says Mother Popped Pills," *Washington Post,* April 30, 1992, https://www.washingtonpost .com/archive/lifestyle/1992/04/30/patti-davis-says-mother-popped-pills /abc9ac5a-7838-41a3-a587-9f6dc32030c6/.

186 **William Rehnquist . . . tranquilizer psychosis:** "FBI Files Detail Rehnquist Drug Addiction," Reuters, January 21, 2007, https://www .reuters.com/article/us-rehnquist-sedatives/fbi-files-detail-rehnquist-drug -addiction-wpost-idUSN0422252220070105.

186 **drug-testing food stamp recipients:** Amanda Michelle Gomez, "What 13 States Discovered After Spending Hundreds of Thousands Drug Testing the Poor," ThinkProgress, April 26, 2019, https://archive .thinkprogress.org/states-cost-drug-screening-testing-tanf-applicants -welfare-2018-results-data-0fe9649fa0f8/.

190 **Despite getting free airtime:** Pamela Warrick, "Can You Just Say No?," *Los Angeles Times,* August 30, 1996, https://www.latimes.com/archives/la -xpm-1996-08-30-ls-38870-story.html.

190 **spending around a million dollars a day:** Ibid.

191 **by its later title, *Reefer Madness*:** Lee, *Smoke Signals,* 52.

193 **largest donors include Purdue Pharma:** Lee Fang, "The Real Reason Pot Is Still Illegal," *The Nation,* July 21, 2014, https://www.thenation.com /article/archive/anti-pot-lobbys-big-bankroll/.

193 **Insys Therapeutics gained FDA approval:** Stacy Lawrence, "Insys to Take On AbbVie with FDA Approval for Oral Cannabinoid," Fierce Biotech, July 5, 2016, https://www.fiercebiotech.com/biotech/insys-to -take-abbvie-fda-approval-for-oral-cannabinoid.

193 **its products in Israeli hospitals:** Javier Hasse, "One of the Largest Pharma Companies in the World Has Made a Big Move in Cannabis," *Forbes*, September 12, 2019, https://www.forbes.com/sites/javierhasse /2019/09/12/big-pharma-teva-cannabis/?sh=6f2e003251f7.

196 **then–Colorado governor John Hickenlooper said:** David Kelly, "Governor Who Called Legalization 'Reckless' Now Says Colorado's Pot Industry Is Working," *Los Angeles Times*, May 17, 2016, https://www .latimes.com/nation/la-na-hickenlooper-marijuana-20160516-20160516 -snap-story.html.

199 **Judy Woodruff, of *PBS NewsHour*, added:** German Lopez, "America's Marijuana Policy Isn't Funny. It's Racist," *Vox*, July 31, 2014, https://www .vox.com/2014/7/31/5952169/marijuana-legalization-jokes-racism.

200 **"Relatively few depictions of marijuana users":** Tara Marie Mortensen et al., "The Marijuana User in US News Media: An Examination of Visual Stereotypes of Race, Culture, Criminality and Normification," *Visual Communication* 19, no. 2 (August 2019), 1, https://journals.sagepub.com /doi/10.1177/1470357219864995.

201 **Carl Sagan, who went on:** Carl Sagan [Mr. X], in *Marihuana Reconsidered*, ed. Lester Grinspoon (Cambridge: Harvard University Press, 1971), 109.

204 **Andrew Weil once said:** Andrew Weil, *The Natural Mind* (Boston: Houghton Mifflin, 1972), 51.

CHAPTER 7: IS RUNNING HIGH ADDICTIVE?

219 **Upton Sinclair line:** Upton Sinclair, *I Candidate for Governor and How I Got Licked* (Berkeley: University of California Press, 1935), 109.

221 **two CU Boulder students served:** Brooke Way, "CU Students Arrested for Feeding Marijuana Brownies to Unassuming Class," Fox 31 News, December 9, 2012, https://kdvr.com/news/2-cu-boulder-students -arrested-after-giving-marijuana-brownies-to-class/.

222 **deaths have climbed 78 percent among men:** Susan Spillane, "Trends in Alcohol-Induced Deaths in the United States, 2000–2016," JAMA Network, February 2020, https://jamanetwork.com/journals /jamanetworkopen/fullarticle/2761545.

225 **Dean was running for the Democratic presidential:** Anne Wallace Allen, "Howard Dean, Once Anti-Pot, Joins Cannabis Company Board,"

VTDigger, April 14, 2019, https://vtdigger.org/2019/04/14/howard-dean
-anti-pot-joins-cannabis-company-board/.

226 **When *Pitchfork* asked:** Jason Crock, "Wilco," *Pitchfork*, May 7, 2007,
https://pitchfork.com/features/interview/6602-wilco/.

227 **behaviors that we consider virtuous:** David J. Linden, *The Compass of
Pleasure* (New York: Penguin, 2011), 25.

227 **"Does this make exercise a virtue":** Ibid., 150.

229 **sugar may be just as addictive as cocaine:** Anna Schaefer and Kareem
Yasin, "Experts Agree: Sugar Might Be as Addictive as Cocaine,"
Healthline, April 30, 2020, https://www.healthline.com/health/food
-nutrition/experts-is-sugar-addictive-drug.

230 **Consumed by 90 percent of American adults:** Diane C. Mitchell,
"Beverage Caffeine Intakes in the U.S.," *Food and Chemical Toxicology* 63
(January 2014), https://www.sciencedirect.com/science/article/pii
/S0278691513007175.

230 **consume it at a rate of 75 percent:** David C. Rettew, "Consider Caffeine
Effects on Children and Adolescents," *MD Edge*, January 14, 2019, https://
www.mdedge.com/pediatrics/article/192652/mental-health/consider
-caffeine-effects-children-and-adolescents.

231 **"Young people have been lied to":** Hunter S. Thompson, *Gonzo: The Life
and Work of Hunter S. Thompson*, directed by Alex Gibney (HDNet Films,
2008), documentary.

238 **much higher success rate:** Hudson Reddon, "Frequent Cannabis Use
and Cessation of Injection of Opioids, Vancouver, Canada, 2005–2018,"
American Journal of Public Health (October 2020), https://pubmed.ncbi
.nlm.nih.gov/32816538/.

240 **35 percent of caffeine users:** Catherine L. W. Striley, "Evaluating
Dependence Criteria for Caffeine," *Journal of Caffeine Research*
(December 2011), https://www.ncbi.nlm.nih.gov/pmc/articles
/PMC3621326/.

242 **"some temporary pleasure":** John Tierney, "The Rational Choices of
Crack Addicts," *New York Times*, September 16, 2013, https://www.ny
times.com/2013/09/17/science/the-rational-choices-of-crack-addicts.html.

EPILOGUE: PROMISES TO KEEP, AND MILES TO GO BEFORE WE SLEEP

278 **binge drinking in states with legal cannabis:** Zoe M. Alley, "Trends in
College Students' Alcohol, Nicotine, Prescription Opioid and Other Drug
Use After Recreational Marijuana Legalization: 2008–2018," *Addictive*

Behaviors (March 2020), https://www.sciencedirect.com/science/article/abs/pii/S030646031930783X.

278 **vehicle fatalities have actually *decreased*:** Collin Calvert, "An Examination of Relationships Between Cannabis Legalization and Fatal Motor Vehicle and Pedestrian-Involved Crashes," *Traffic Injury Prevention* (2020), https://pubmed.ncbi.nlm.nih.gov/32856949/.

278 **more of a success than a failure:** Linley Sanders, "States with Marijuana Legalization View the Legislation as a Success," YouGov, May 13, 2020, https://today.yougov.com/topics/economy/articles-reports/2020/05/13/recreational-marijuana-poll?.

279 **making up 45 percent of the population:** Paul Schwartzman and John D. Harden, "D.C. Legalized Marijuana, but One Thing Didn't Change: Almost Everyone Arrested on Pot Charges Is Black," *Washington Post*, September 15, 2020, https://www.washingtonpost.com/local/legal-issues/dc-marijuana-arrest-legal/2020/09/15/65c20348-d01b-11ea-9038-af089b63ac21_story.html.

280 **4 percent of the cannabis market ownership:** Nick Charles, "Black Entrepreneurs Struggle to Join Legal Weed Industry," NBC News, February 11, 2020, https://www.nbcnews.com/news/nbcblk/black-entrepreneurs-struggle-join-legal-weed-industry-n1132351.

280 **$70 to $130 billion:** Eli McVey, "Chart: US Cannabis Industry's Economic Impact Could Hit $130 Billion by 2024," *Marijuana Business Daily*, July 21, 2020, https://mjbizdaily.com/chart-us-cannabis-industrys-economic-impact-could-hit-130-billion-by-2024/.

INDEX

INDEX

INDEX